"*Apothecary Cocktails* is crafted like one of Warren's libations, creative, beautiful, well balanced, and delicious! A staple for any home bar."

—GABLE ERENZO, distiller, brand ambassador, Tuthilltown Spirits (Gardiner, NY)

"There's no doubt about the restorative power of a good cocktail after a bad day. Warren Bobrow builds on this motif, serving up a collection of creative drink recipes alongside historical anecdotes and lush, thirst-inducing photographs."

—KARA NEWMAN, author, *Cocktails for a Crowd*

"Warren gets to the heart of the fact that drinking was once as much about being restorative and curative as it was for pleasure. The happy coincidence of the two is wonderfully illustrated here."

—ROCKY YEH, cocktail visionary, bartender, Vessel (Seattle, WA)

"In *Apothecary Cocktails*, Warren gives us all permission to live and drink well. Stock full of recipes dripping in delicious bitters and healthful herbs, take the plunge with this book and learn how Warren's enticing cocktails will keep you healthier and happier."

—SUZANNE LONG, mixologist, Mixanthrope.com

"Warren Bobrow delivers to the reader what many cocktail books promise but fail to deliver—a clear, uncomplicated path to satisfying drinks based on a bit of the history behind the libation."

—EDWARD HAMILTON, creator of the Ministry of Rum blog and author of *Rums of the Eastern Caribbean* and *The Complete Guide to Rum*

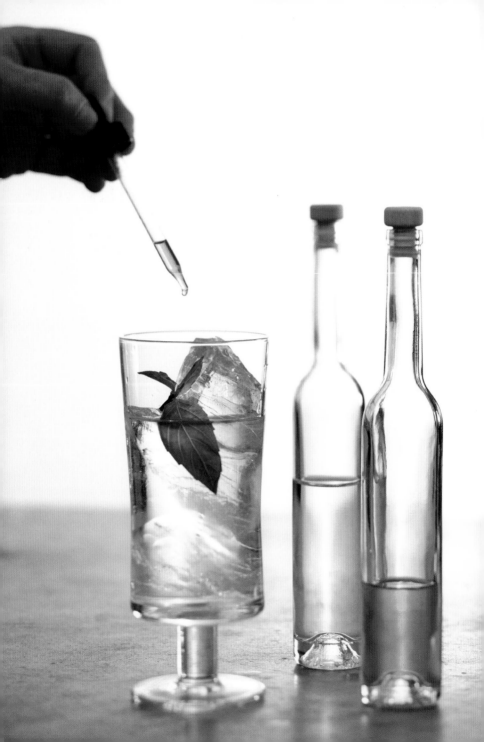

Apothecary Cocktails

RESTORATIVE DRINKS
from YESTERDAY *and* TODAY

WARREN BOBROW

FAIR WINDS
PRESS
BEVERLY, MASSACHUSETTS

Dedication
To my wife, Julie, who suggested I become a writer in the first place.

First published in the USA in 2013 by
Fair Winds Press, a member of
Quayside Publishing Group
100 Cummings Center
Suite 406-L
Beverly, MA 01915-6101
www.fairwindspress.com
Visit www.QuarrySPOON.com and help us celebrate food and culture
one spoonful at a time!

17 16 15 14 13   2 3 4 5

ISBN: 978-1-59233-584-8

Digital edition published in 2013
eISBN: 978-1-61058-859-1

Library of Congress Cataloging-in-Publication Data available

Cover and book design by Kathie Alexander
Photography by Glenn Scott Photography

Printed and bound in China

The information in this book is for educational purposes only.
It is not intended to replace the advice of a physician or medical practitioner.
Please see your health care provider before beginning any new health program.

Foreword

nce you meet Warren Bobrow, it doesn't take long
to realize that he's been bitten by the bug. In 2009,
after spending more than twenty years in corporate
America, Warren tossed aside a successful career in
the banking industry to pursue his passion for the
culinary and cocktail world. Over the past three years, Warren
has not only redefined himself as an individual, but also he has
explored the world of food and drink from a unique perspective;
he has shared his journey with his readers in hundreds of articles published in magazines, encyclopedias, and blogs globally.
In *Apothecary Cocktails: Restorative Drinks from Yesterday and
Today*, Warren will both inform and entertain you as he nego-
tiates the history of pre-Prohibition cocktails, bitters, tinctures,
and tonics from the apothecaries of days gone by.

When I first met Warren in 2011, I was impressed and delighted
by his passion for writing, eating, and drinking. *Apothecary
Cocktails: Restorative Drinks from Yesterday and Today* is
destined to become a classic for both seasoned and aspiring
bartenders and cocktail enthusiasts around the world.

A hearty toast to Warren and Apothecary Cocktails*!*

Paul G. Tuennerman (a.k.a. Mr. Cocktail)
Co-Owner, Tales of the Cocktail

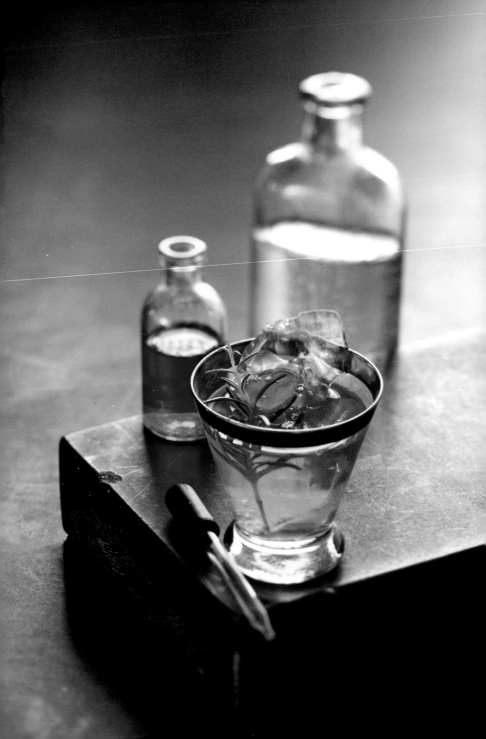

Contents

Introduction
From Old-Time Apothecaries to Contemporary Cocktails:
A Brief History of Herbal Healing 8

Introduction

From Old-Time Apothecaries to Contemporary Cocktails:
A Brief History of Herbal Healing

pothecary cocktails have a rich and intriguing history. As their name suggests, these curative cocktails were originally created in early pharmacies or apothecaries, from ancient times until the beginning of the twentieth century. I've been interested in the history of patent medicines and apothecaries for as long as I can remember. My grandfather was in the patent pharmaceutical business and, even as a child, the world of patent medicines and quack cures were a part of my day-to-day life. In fact, they were impossible to ignore, because I was fed a teaspoon of spirit-based vitamin tonic along with my chewable vitamins and orange juice at breakfast every day. (I think I turned out pretty well, despite having consumed a daily teaspoon of 50-proof spirits first thing in the morning during my tender years.) Being exposed to these combinations of herbs and spices with alcohol early in life—a little too early, arguably—led to my interests in mixology and the apothecary cocktail movement as an adult.

Like most apothecaries of yesteryear, I'm not a doctor, but I am interested in healing through natural, herb-based methods. Before the advent of modern medicine, ordinary people had minimal access to qualified doctors, so early pharmacists acted as local medical professionals to the sick in their communities. Because doctors didn't manufacture medicines themselves, it fell to the pharmacist to prescribe, create, and administer healing potions to their patients (usually in very small, carefully measured amounts). They manufactured tinctures, bitters, elixirs, and tonics for all kinds of ailments; using primitive ingredients, some of these recipes were old as spoken history. These healing, homemade potions may have been laced with copious amounts of distilled alcohol, then stirred or shaken before being poured directly into a glass and given to the patient on the spot as a prescriptive. The earliest known pharmacist-prepared treatments called for fragile herbs, flowers, fruits, and even vegetables—along with the aforementioned substantial quantities of alcohol, which prevented them from rotting, and preserved their healing qualities. Most of these botanicals would have been grown right in the apothecaries' own kitchen gardens to ensure freshness and potency. Each formulary would have been custom made, depending on the individual patient's complaint, and was hand-prepared from start to finish.

It's true that not every cure was strictly successful. Before medicine was standardized, the early pharmacist would have been part carnival barker, part folk doctor, part surgeon, and part snake-oil purveyor. However, this is not to say that every apothecary traded in pseudo-cures: many, even most, pharmacists were very serious about their calling as healers. But in the absence of medical doctors, their patients would have called upon them to cure just about anything, from stomachaches to mood swings to infected wounds. Occasionally, pharmacists were even expected to perform complex medical tasks, such as surgeries, with minimal equipment and supplies. In short, an awful lot was demanded of them.

Most importantly, a successful pharmacist had to earn his customers' trust, and that meant delivering curatives that would actually work. Many of the most effective curatives in the United States were introduced by immigrants from Europe, Asia, and the Caribbean islands, who brought some of their healing methods (and their exotic ingredients) with them. Folk treatments using herbs suspended in alcohol had been commonplace in all of these locations for hundreds of years, so the methods these immigrant healers practiced would have dated back centuries—if not millennia. These treatments included alcoholic bitters, which I use frequently in the recipes in this book. Bitters are highly concentrated herbal concoctions that were prescribed to treat a multitude of afflictions, including malaises of the stomach and respiratory systems. Like their European counterparts, American pharmacists came to view them as reliable curatives—especially in the absence of modern pharmaceutical companies that could produce and distribute synthetic drugs.

> "Consulting your local mixologist about a healing cocktail is not far removed from the way in which patients would have approached their local pharmacist in years past."

Technology sufficient to manufacture drugs safely, and in large quantities, hadn't yet been created, so curatives like bitters became absorbed into American healing practices. In fact, it wasn't until the nineteenth century that drugs would be available across the country.

In New Orleans in 1816, Louis Dufilho became the first licensed pharmacist in the United States. As a new law ruled, his apothecary shop was permitted to both compound and sell formularies for healing. Dufilho developed quite a clientele, who frequented his pharmacy to obtain both alcoholic and nonalcoholic curatives. It wasn't until 1906, when the Pure Food and Drug Act was passed, that the government became involved in maintaining the purity of apothecary-produced curatives. Subsequently, the Pure Food and Drug Act, which would later become the U.S. Food and Drug Administration (FDA), moved alcohol-based "cocktails" and other curative preparations involving alcohol out of the pharmacies and into the cocktail bar, where they have remained ever since. Many modern types of liquor are distilled with naturally derived ingredients—minus the narcotics that would've appeared in them in the past!

These days, drinkers are more interested in the ingredients and the lore of apothecary-inspired cocktails, and don't necessarily visit cocktail bars to be cured of an illness. Instead, they're enthralled by the histories of many older brands of liquors, some of which were originally created to be medicines or tonics. And they appreciate the use of herbal ingredients that would have been apothecary staples back in the day. This revival and reinterpretation of antique methods of healing reflects the fact that twenty-first century tipplers are trying to eat and drink more healthfully—and more authentically. To fill these demands, a major resurgence of farm- or garden-to-bar "gartenders" has popped up—professionals who go much further than merely adding a slice of citrus or a purée of bland tomatoes to their cocktail creations. These creative healers research traditional apothecary methods, sometimes tracking down long-lost ingredients, to re-create the cocktails of the past. They use fresh herbs, vegetables, bitters, and liqueurs that were created as digestives in their mixology—just as their predecessors, the early apothecaries, did.

Cocktail bars with an emphasis on the apothecary, such as Apotheke in New York City, have sprung up around the country. And it makes sense: Consulting your local mixologist about a healing cocktail is not far removed from the way in which patients would have approached their local pharmacist in years past. Just as customers today visit their local bars or cocktail lounges seeking a wise, friendly bartender who'll listen to their troubles, patients would visit apothecaries to discuss curatives for their ills. These consultations would take place in private, in a room adjacent to the pharmacy—making the client-apothecary relationship a very personal one.

This book takes its inspiration from that relationship. As early pharmacists would have done when preparing prescriptives for their patients, it privileges fresh ingredients, using a wide variety of herbs, fruits, and vegetables, all of which have been specially selected for their healing elements. Whether you're after a stomach-soothing digestif, a little of the hair of the dog that bit you, or a steaming-hot concoction to warm you during the winter months, there's a delicious, medicinal cocktail for everyone in the seventy-five recipes I've chosen. Although the cocktails in this book aren't meant to replace medicine, I hope they'll make you as eager as I am to recreate the apothecary cocktails of yesterday in your own kitchen.

Warren Bobrow

Note for the Reader:

All recipes make a single serving, unless otherwise indicated.
All herbs are fresh, unless otherwise indicated.

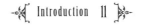

1 Digestives and Other Curatives
Soothers and Libations for All That Ails You

he stomach is a sensitive creature. Heavy meals can stress it out; a bout of the flu can send it into serious distress; motion sickness might make it turn cartwheels; and a case of the nerves has been known to send it into SOS mode. And according to Murphy's Law—which states that anything that can go wrong, will, and at the worst possible time—you can bet that your belly will mutiny just when you need it to be on its best behavior.

Believe it or not, it's likely that our forefathers had it even worse. In the eighteenth and nineteenth centuries, when home refrigerators were only the stuff of dreams, it was difficult to preserve food and prevent it from spoiling. Plus, kitchen cleanliness wasn't what it is nowadays, and modern preventative measures, such as antibiotics and flu shots, had yet to be discovered. This means indigestion, bellyaches, food poisoning, and other belly-related maladies were common occurrences—and apothecaries had to be well-stocked with remedies for the ill-tempered tummy.

And they certainly had plenty to work with. With the help of local botanicals, pharmacists would mix herbal tinctures and tonics that could alleviate nausea and stomach pain, and suspend the mixtures in doses of alcohol to keep them fresh. These curatives were available only at the apothecary's shop, and their recipes were usually closely guarded. Tinctures like these were the forerunners of digestifs that are still enjoyed around the world today, such as Chartreuse, Fernet Branca, amaro, and Bénédictine. Usually taken after dinner to ease stomachs suffering from too much good food and drink, these liqueurs often have a bracingly bitter flavor from the wide variety of herbs used to produce them.

Other liquors, too, were created to relieve digestive disorders. The famous (or, perhaps, infamous) tipple absinthe contained the belly benefiting leaves and blossoms of the wormwood plant—and blamed for the allegedly psychedelic effects that the absinthe produced in drinkers. Wormwood was also added to vermouth, which was taken neat to calm bellies: In fact, vermouth was said to be able to detoxify the body and, according to legend, could even alleviate or prevent food poisoning. Brandy found its way into a number of stomach cures, since it was thought to be a powerful laxative and purgative. Apothecaries prescribed it in the hopes that it would quickly eliminate harmful toxins in instances of poisoning. (It was even used to treat recovering opium addicts after an initial purge using vinegar and water.) Aromatic bitters, which are related to herbal liquors like Italian amari, would have been used liberally in curatives, or taken on their own with a dash of fizzy water to calm edgy stomachs.

Of course, potent liquors and bitter herbs weren't the only stomach-soothing ingredients an apothecary would've had at his disposal. Garden vegetables, such as rhubarb and fennel, could also help relieve stomach ailments. Rhubarb (the stems, not the leaves: rhubarb leaves are toxic) is also an effective laxative, and has been used to promote good digestion for centuries. Fragrant, crunchy, anise-flavored fennel, too, is good for the belly: Consumed raw or taken as a herbal tea, apothecaries would've championed it to those who had overindulged in their victuals. Aniseed and star anise were also used for all things alimentary, in both traditional Chinese and Western medicine—that's why the Italian digestive, sambuca, has such a distinctive aniseed taste.

> "Pharmacists of yesteryear would also have worked household staples into their curatives. A nice hot cup of tea is said to be a quick cure for ailments of the spirit, and makes troubles seem more manageable."

Pharmacists of yesteryear would also have worked household staples into their curatives. A nice hot cup of tea is said to be a quick cure for ailments of the spirit, and makes troubles seem more manageable—but tea could also be used to deliver warming, healing ingredients, including herbs and alcohol, to a patient complaining of an upset stomach. Sparkling waters, such as club soda, seltzer water, and quinine-rich tonic water, often top off stomach-soothing libations, or could even bring relief on their own. Their effervescence can refresh tired palates, and seem to make all the difference when it comes to indigestion. (Somehow, bubbles make everything better.)

This chapter shows you how to put those bubbles to good use. You'll be refreshed by cocktails such as the *Peppery Fennel Fizz*, a spicy, healing combination of the Turkish liqueur raki, a fennel-infused simple syrup, dried chile, and orange bitters, which can't help but give sluggish digestion a boost. If it's hotter than hot outside, blitz up a batch of *Rhubarb Slushies*: they're made sans fizzy water, but they're magical concoctions of rhubarb tea liqueur, a delicate rose-infused simple syrup, and plenty of crushed ice. Or, if you're a bit overstuffed after dinner, look no further than the Vieux *Carré Cocktail*: it administers healing draughts of Bénédictine, vermouth, and rye whiskey, along with stomach-friendly bitters, and does it in style. For a twist on the classic rum and cola, try replacing the rum with *Fernet Branca* for an Italian-inspired digestif that'll destress any belly—or reach for a *Sazerac Cocktail*, an old-fashioned combination of rye whiskey, simple syrup, bitters, and just a hint of absinthe. Read on for many more delicious ways to banish bellyaches—and fast.

Note for the Reader:

All recipes make a single serving, unless otherwise indicated.
All herbs are fresh, unless otherwise indicated.

Fernet Branca and Cola

When it comes to mangia e beve *(eat and drink), few cultures can surpass the delights of Italy. And there's little better after a sumptuous meal than a nip of the Italian herbal liqueur Fernet Branca, which sports an assertive, even bitter flavor that's truly inimitable. This historic cocktail actually hails from Argentina, where Fernet Branca remains popular with the families of Italian immigrants who left their homeland during World War II. Don't be afraid of Fernet's bitter edge: When served in a cocktail alongside cane-sugar cola, this deeply engaging elixir acts as a soothing finish to a heavy meal. The body-warming alcohol levels of the liqueur also play a role in the intense flavor of the naturally sourced herbs and spices. Fernet Branca is delicious when taken ice cold, as is the custom in Argentina and San Francisco, with a tall glass of cola on the side.*

---

2 ounces (60 ml) Fernet Branca

Ice cubes

4 ounces (120 ml) cane-sugar cola (or regular cola)

¼ lime, cut into chunks

Pour the measure of Fernet Branca over a handful of ice cubes in a tall Collins glass. Top with the cane-sugar cola, and add a chunk or two of lime to give the immune system a boost (it rarely hurts to add citrus to curative cocktails). Your stomach—and head—will thank you after one of these calming digestifs. ↷

Fernet Branca with English Breakfast Tea and Raw Honey

Fernet Branca was invented in nineteenth-century Italy to ease maladies of the belly, and it's certainly retained its marketing mystique, even a century and a half later. Fernet is certainly easy to quaff on its own or mixed with cola—but it's just as good served steaming hot. In the Caribbean, it's often paired with English breakfast tea and honey, a combination that's said to relieve stomachaches of all sorts (including those caused by spending too much time in the sun sipping cocktails, perhaps?). Plus, as any apothecary of auld lang syne would have agreed, both warm liquids and honey can aid digestion. Nota bene: While it calls for English breakfast tea, the Cocktail Whisperer doesn't recommend trying this curative for breakfast. You've been warned.

3 ounces (90 ml) Fernet Branca

Pot of strong English breakfast tea (about 2 cups [475 ml])

2 tablespoons (40 g) raw honey

Preheat two mugs by filling them with boiling water; discard the water after a few seconds. Add 1½ ounces (45 ml) of Fernet Branca to each mug. Fill the mugs with tea, and stir a tablespoon (20 g) of honey into each mug. Lean back, sip slowly, and let the healing begin. Serves 2.

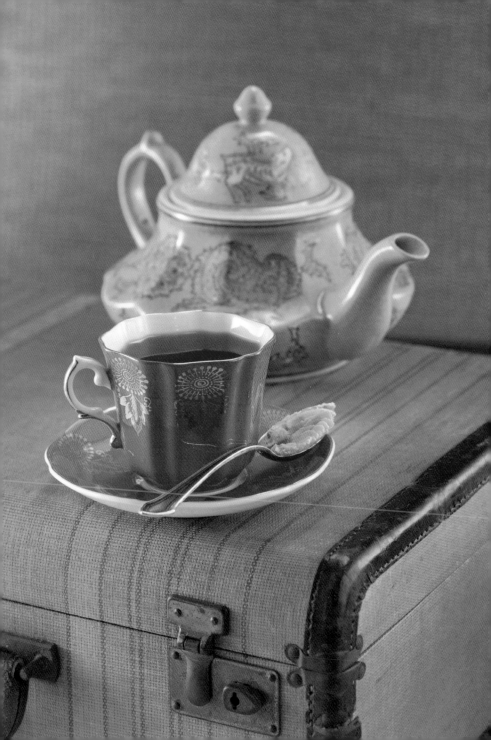

Sazerac Cocktail

Created in New Orleans early in the twentieth century, the Sazerac Cocktail still occupies a well-deserved spot in our cabinet of healing cocktails. It calls for Peychaud's bitters, a New Orleans–based brand that was originally intended to heal stomach sicknesses, as well as the infamous liqueur, absinthe—also known as the Green Fairy or La Fée Verte, due to its bright-green hue. Back in the day, the wormwood in absinthe would have placed this cocktail as a curative, since it was reputed to be both an antispasmodic and a digestive aid. (Licorice-scented anisette is a good replacement for absinthe if you can't find it.) This version of the Sazerac calls for rye whiskey instead of traditional cognac, and it's a powerfully sweet, strikingly colorful, and deliciously healing reminder of the apothecary days of the past.

---

1 ounce (30 ml) absinthe (or anisette)

2½ ounces (75 ml) rye whiskey

4 tablespoons (60 ml) simple syrup (see page 155)

Ice cubes

Several dashes of Peychaud's bitters

2 lemon twists

Wash two rocks glasses with the absinthe by pouring ½ ounce (15 ml) absinthe into each glass, swirling it around, and pouring it out—preferably into your mouth! Divide the rye whiskey between the two glasses. Add 2 tablespoons (30 ml) of simple syrup to each glass. Pop 1 large ice cube into each cocktail, and top each with a dash or two of bitters. Garnish the drinks with lemon twists. Lift your glasses high, and drink to happier bellies. Serves 2. ❧

Chartreuse Elixir Application

The legendary Chartreuse Vegetal Elixir is not imported into the United States—and perhaps for good reason, since its alcohol content approaches a blistering 140 proof. (Feel free to substitute regular chartreuse for this recipe instead.) Chartreuse contains over 130 herbs, but the recipe is guarded as if it were the Holy Grail: Produced in the French Alps by the Péres Chartreux monks, the mystical powers of the ingredients are guarded so closely that only three monks at a time are trusted with the original recipe for the Chartreuse Vegetal Elixir. Although the monks only produce a small amount of the liqueur today, Chartreuse Vegetal Elixir is sold in the same liquid form today as it was originally distilled, and is best served straight from a teaspoon or dripped onto a sugar cube to balance its bitter flavor. The Péres Chartreux monks believe that the key to their long life is facilitated through the careful—and regular—application of these potent herbal ingredients.

---

1 teaspoon Chartreuse Vegetal Elixir (or Chartreuse VEP—that is, chartreuse aged for an exceptionally long time)

1 sugar cube

Dash of seltzer water, about ¼ ounce (7 ml)

Using a teaspoon, slowly drip the chartreuse onto a sugar cube. Place the sugar cube in your mouth, under the tongue, if desired, until dissolved. Or, place the chartreuse-soaked sugar cube into a bit of seltzer water, and muddle to a soft paste with a cocktail stick.

Top with a bit more seltzer and drink quickly to good health. A spoonful of sugar really does help the medicine go down. ↝

The Iberville Street Cocktail

The Iberville Street Cocktail, a tasty variation on the Sazerac theme, would have been just as effective as the Sazerac against tummy troubles—mostly due to the generous use of those healing Peychaud's bitters, which coat the inside of the stomach. French-born pharmacist Antoine Peychaud developed his recipe for bitters in 1830—long before safe food-handling practices became de rigueur—to relieve stomach illnesses of the era. His soothing recipe contained anise, cloves, cinnamon, and nutmeg, along with copious amounts of brandy. For a time, Peychaud's combination of herbs, spices, and alcohol were available only in pharmacies, and were even meant to ease the symptoms of more serious diseases, such as dysentery and ulcers. Today, luckily, you don't need a prescription to make an Iberville, which includes absinthe, brandy for tension relief, and grapefruit juice for a hit of healing citrus.

2 ounces (60 ml) Lillet Blanc

1 ounce (30 ml) brandy

4-5 dashes of Peychaud's bitters

4 ounces (120 ml) freshly squeezed grapefruit juice

½ ounce (15 ml) absinthe

Large piece of lemon peel

1 orange zest twist

Ice

Add a couple handfuls of ice to a Boston shaker; then add the Lillet Blanc, brandy, bitters, and grapefruit juice, and shake well for twenty seconds.

Wash a short rocks glass with the absinthe by pouring the absinthe into the glass, swirling it around, and pouring it out. Rub the inside of the washed glass thoroughly with the lemon peel. Strain the stomach-healing mixture into the glass, and garnish with a flamed orange zest twist (hold the orange twist firmly behind a lit match, and pinch it to release its natural citrus oils). Sip slowly for quick relief of uneasy stomachs. ⌒𝄐

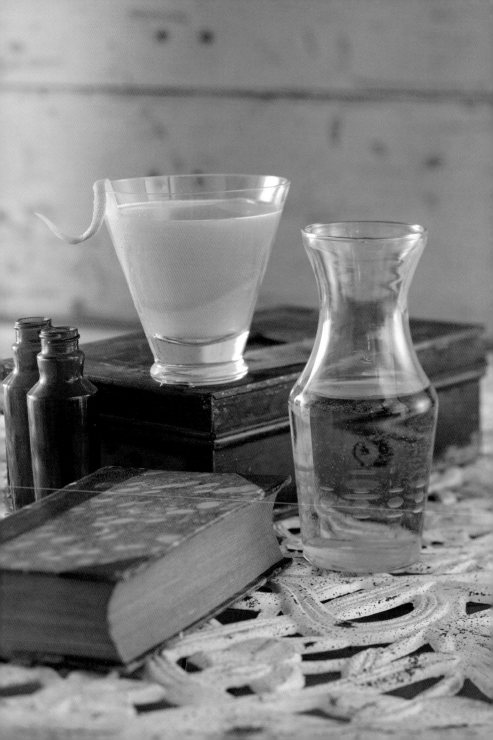

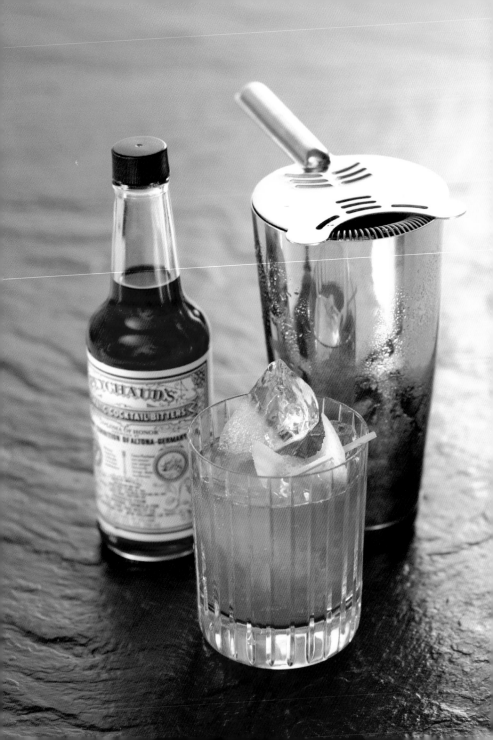

Vieux Carré Cocktail

The herb-based liqueur Bénédictine was developed with the aid of a pharmacist in eighteenth-century France. Boasting twenty-seven herbs and exotic spices suspended in an alcohol base, Bénédictine was created as a tonic for stimulating the circulatory system. In later years, it was found to aid in the digestion of the notoriously butter- and cream-laden French cooking of days gone by. Bénédictine is still sold on its own, but it's also available on the American market under the name "B&B," blended with brandy. But you don't have to confine Bénédictine to your brandy snifter. The healing Vieux Carré Cocktail combines Bénédictine with rye whiskey, absinthe, cognac, Peychaud's bitters, and that famous stomach curative, Angostura bitters, into an elixir that dates back to an original recipe from the historic Hotel Monteleone in New Orleans, where treating the sick with carefully concocted, alcoholic curatives was the order of the day.

1 ounce (30 ml) rye whiskey

1 ounce (30 ml) cognac

1 ounce (30 ml) sweet vermouth

2 to 3 shakes Peychaud's bitters

2 to 3 shakes Angostura bitters

½ ounce (15 ml) Bénédictine

Lemon zest twist

Ice

Add the rye whiskey, cognac, vermouth, bitters, and Bénédictine to a mixing glass over a couple handfuls of ice. Mix well, then strain into a short rocks glass. Twist the lemon zest over the edge of the glass. Stomach malaise, be gone! ☙

Bénédictine Twist Elixir

The herb angelica, which is used in the production of Bénédictine, chartreuse, gin, and vermouth, has been used as a natural stimulant for hundreds of years, and has been said to relieve illnesses of the respiratory and digestive systems. And this elixir is just the thing when it comes to rousing the digestion after an especially rich meal. With its haunting note of exotic spices and deeply aromatic Bénédictine, it tastes just medicinal enough to convince you that the liqueur is doing its healing work, and doing it well. There's no better digestif than the Bénédictine Twist Elixir, which adds a splash of fizzy water and lemon zest twists to the potent liqueur to perk up an overworked palate. (Don't skip the lemon twists: a dose of citrus is always a great idea when it comes to curative cocktails like this one.)

2 ounces (60 ml) Bénédictine

2 to 3 lemon zest twists

Ice cube

1 to 2 ounces (30 to60 ml) seltzer water

Add the Bénédictine and the lemon zest twists to a snifter glass. Pop one large ice cube into the glass, and top with the seltzer water. Serve a round as a last course at your next dinner party. Your guests are sure to head home with happy bellies. ➷

Habsburg Stomach Healer

In 1790, Dr. József Zwack, the royal physician to the Habsburg Court, developed a medicinal blend of forty herbs and spices intended to soothe the stomach and prevent illnesses of all sorts. This tonic-based apothecary liqueur is still produced today according to the same recipe. It calls for macerated and distilled herbs to be aged in specially sourced oak casks, which add color, flavor, and depth to this bitter Hungarian health tonic. Said to be a powerful detoxifier, Zwack is enjoyed both as an aperitif and a digestif, and it's usually administered straight up and well chilled (according to some, adding ice would only dilute and weaken the effects of the potent liqueur). For the faint of heart, though, it can be mixed with ice and seltzer or tonic water: hence, the Habsburg Stomach Healer. Try to find a tonic water made with cane sugar; it's far superior to the run-of-the-mill stuff.

---

2 ounces (60 ml) Zwack

3 ounces (90 ml) cane sugar
tonic water

Ice

Four drops of curry bitters

Fill a Collins glass with ice. Pour the Zwack over the ice, and top with tonic water. Add the bitters, and mix gently. Sip slowly, and let the Zwack work its medicinal magic. ❧

Root and Rye

The original Rock and Rye cocktail, a mixture of rye whiskey, simple syrup, and citrus fruits, was a nineteenth- and twentieth-century classic. The simple concoction was believed to be a cure for chest congestion, stubborn coughs, and even the common cold. This delicious spin on the Rock and Rye calls for a special ingredient that tips its hat to the early era of medicinal folk healers. It's called root tea, but it's not the kind of tea you'd drink alongside your breakfast bagel. Based on a recipe that's said to have been handed down by Native Americans to pre-colonial settlers, root tea liqueur is a spirit that's been developed to imitate the original flavors and healing techniques of the early apothecary age, using natural materials such as birch bark, sassafras, anise, and cloves. Thanks to root tea liqueur, the Root and Rye gently becalms uneasy bellies, and is especially refreshing on hot summer days.

---

1 ounce (30 ml) organic root tea liqueur

2 ounces (60 ml) rye whiskey

1 rock candy swizzle stick

6 ounces (175 ml) sarsaparilla or birch beer

Ice

Pack a tall Collins glass with ice. Add the root tea liqueur and the rye whiskey, followed by the sarsaparilla or birch beer. Mix well with the rock candy swizzle stick, sip slowly, and let the Root and Rye settle down that sour stomach. ❧

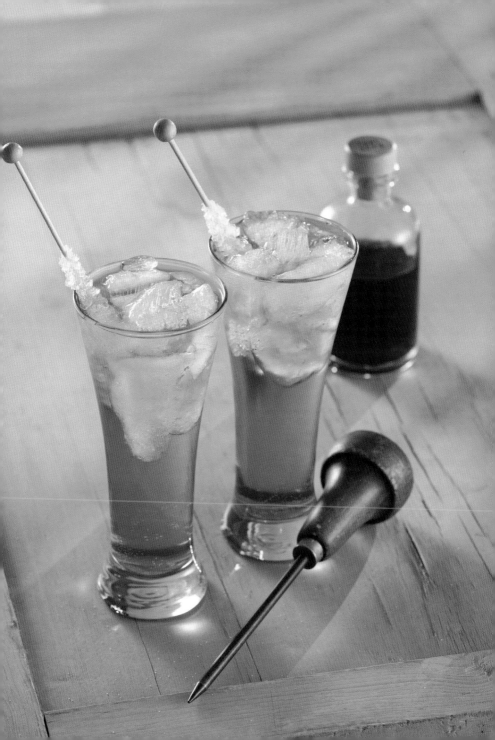

Rhubarb Slushy

Rhubarb has been used in folk medicine for thousands of years, and, legend has it, first arrived in the United States when Benjamin Franklin brought rhubarb seeds from Europe in the late eighteenth century. Famed for its powerful purgative qualities, rhubarb has been known to ease blockages of the digestive tract that may stem from poor diet. (And it's rich in vitamin C and potassium, too.) In its incarnation as a liqueur, it's a delicious way to relax stomachs on the fritz. Sure to summon up memories of late summers long past, this grown-up slushy puts rhubarb liqueur into the limelight, combining it with a delicately fragrant simple syrup infused with rose. A dash of bitters tops off this restorative cocktail.

---

3 ounces (90 ml) rhubarb tea liqueur

Crushed ice

2 tablespoons (30 ml) rose-infused simple syrup (see page 157)

Four drops Thai bitters

Pack a Collins glass with the crushed ice. Pour the rhubarb tea liqueur and rose-infused simple syrup over it. Mix well with a bar spoon until combined. Add the Thai bitters. The result will be a fantastically icy, slushy concoction—hence the name—that's best served with a spoon and a straw.

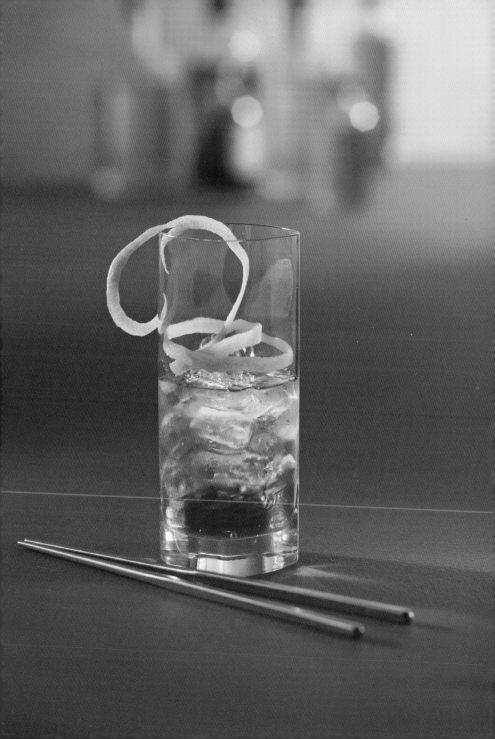

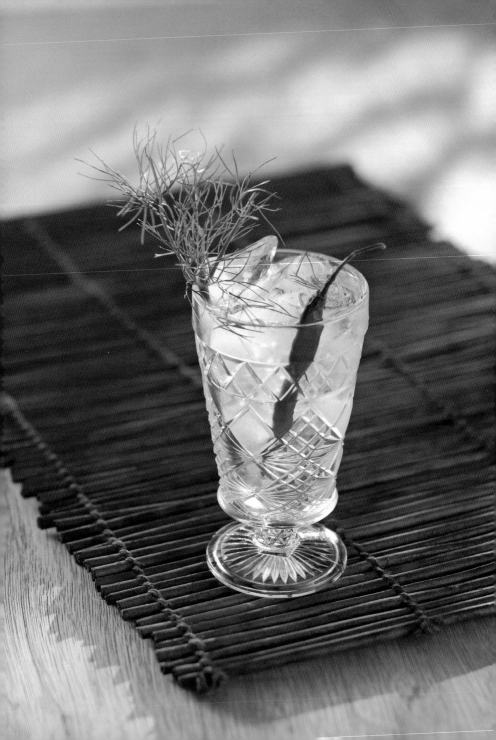

Peppery Fennel Fizz

There's nothing better than a multi-course meal with friends, complete with dessert and drinks—lots of drinks. Of course, your stomach won't always thank you the next day. That's where our friend fennel comes in. It's often used as a diuretic, and is said to remedy digestive malaises of all kinds—plus, it's a powerfully purifying, detoxifying vegetable. It's simple to whip up a cleansing, refreshing cocktail featuring fennel that peps up your palate as well as your belly. Here, fennel syrup is combined with raki, the anise-based Turkish spirit, along with chile flakes, which jolt taste buds back to life (and if the chile makes you sweat a bit, so much the better.) And the effervescence in a dose of seltzer water helps to settle overworked stomachs, too.

---

1 ounce (30 ml) fennel simple syrup (see page 155)

2 ounces (60 ml) raki or absinthe

¼ teaspoon dried chile flakes

1 teaspoon orange bitters

4 ounces (120 ml) seltzer water

Ice

Fill a tall Collins glass with crushed ice. Add the fennel simple syrup, raki, chile flakes, and bitters—use the full teaspoon, don't skimp! Stir gently, top with seltzer water, sip, and let the detox begin. ↷

2 Winter Warmers ⟩⟩

Drinks to Chase the Chill Away

here's a lot to love about winter. Its crisp, bracing weather leaves you ruddy-cheeked and glowing; the party-packed holiday season, with all of its bustle and fun (not to mention delicious food and drink) is a dose of good cheer for the spirit; and wintery sports like skiing and ice skating come into their own once again. And it's just the right time to enjoy well-made cocktails—especially those that can warm you from the inside out.

Healing, warming winter drinks are great remedies for that deep-down, seeps-way-into-your-bones kind of cold. They're not just designed to provide a few minutes of penetrating heat to stiff fingers; they're meant to warm chilly bodies for hours at a time. Apothecaries of old would have had a thorough knowledge of the effects of cold weather upon the body—and would have been well versed in how to treat those effects. In colder climates, such as the northernmost reaches of the United States, curatives for serious chills abound. Originally, winter warmers such as these would have had roots in other countries well known for their frosty weather during the long winter months, such as Denmark, Norway, Sweden, Russia, and the Ukraine. In regions such as these, it's not just the low temperatures that make the cold difficult to bear; it's also the lack of sunlight, which makes winter days nearly as dark as winter nights, and can lead to sluggishness and sinking spirits. It's not surprising, then, that the pharmacies in

Scandinavian countries carry many varieties of herbal elixirs, bitters, and tonics—many of them are based on special combinations of botanicals that are specifically designed to warm the body from within. Some of these elixirs can be combined with liquids that are already hot, such as strong, black tea, stimulating coffee, or thick, bone-warming soups for double the chill-fighting power.

As apothecaries of old knew well, a single cure can treat a variety of maladies. The ingredients in warming winter cocktails do more than just counteract the cold. The delicious, healing Slavic soup borscht uses fresh beets as its base. Beets are a good source of vitamins and antioxidants and have been used since Roman times as an aphrodisiac and as a remedy for digestive disorders. Citrus fruits and their juices are powerful assets to the immune system, as sailors of days gone by would have known: without precious vitamin C, sailors would have been subject to life-threatening diseases such as scurvy. Everyone loves the warming taste and fragrance of ginger—think gingerbread and other holiday desserts—but it's also an effective antidote to seasickness and nausea. Plus, tasty, frost-battling winter warmers need not be highly alcoholic to banish the chills—although a little liquor certainly helps! Feel free to tinker with the amount of alcohol in the drinks in this chapter if you're a less-is-more type of tippler.

Too Much of a Good Thing

Do you remember going skiing with a flask of hot cocoa in your pocket liberally corrected with intoxicating liquor for a quick blast of warming heat directly through your veins? Well, if you like that instant feeling of warmth, these winter warmers will warm you from the inside out. Please keep in mind, however, that too much alcohol in freezing weather can result in your complete inability to feel the cold. That can lead to frost-bitten extremities! Drink gently and keep yourself bundled up!

"After a day spent on the slopes, relax in front of the fire with the Mountain Body Warmer, which combines a pungent German schnapps with refreshing, hydrating herbal tea for a pick-me-up that lasts all afternoon."

The drinks in this chapter have been created to nourish and thaw shivery bodies, and to restore numbed spirits. After a day spent on the slopes, relax in front of the fire with the *Mountain Body Warmer*, which combines a pungent German schnapps with refreshing, hydrating herbal tea for a pick-me-up that lasts all afternoon. If you crave something more substantial, mix up a batch of *Roasted Beet Borscht with Sour Cream and Vodka*—and marvel at its neon-pink hue! It's a meal in itself, and the vodka provides an extra dose of warmth. Or, opt for a sweet treat: *The Centerba and Chocolate Chaud* suspends a curative dose of the herbal Italian liqueur, Centerba, in a bath of homemade hot chocolate that's perfect after dinner or on snowy afternoons. (This bone-warming concoction is for grownups only, of course—whip up a batch of booze-free hot chocolate for the kids so they don't get jealous.) If Navy-strength healing is what you need, reach for a ration of citrusy grog or hot buttered rum; these rum-based remedies are part of a long seafaring tradition in which sailors had to battle extreme climactic conditions, such as storms and bitter cold, as a matter of course.

If the temperature's plummeted, you're battling the sniffles, and the weather outside is nothing short of frightful, never fear: The delicious, nourishing cocktails in this chapter are sure to keep you warmed through until spring.

Note for the Reader:

All recipes make a single serving, unless otherwise indicated.
All herbs are fresh, unless otherwise indicated.

Mountain Body Warmer

That world-famous herbal (or sometimes fruit-laced) German concentrate of distilled spirits called schnapps delivers rapid inner heating that can counteract the effects of cold and snowy weather. Schnapps—which has been around for centuries, and was originally only available from apothecaries—can also offer much-needed relief from the winter colds and coughs that can ravage the throat and respiratory system. (As the Russian proverb goes, "Drink a glass of schnapps after your soup and you steal a ruble from the doctor.") Germans mix it with hot tea, honey, and lemon; pour it into flasks; and use it to warm both body and mind when outdoors during the chilly months. Mix up a pot of this soothing tea before or after heading outdoors in wintertime; you'll feel refreshed by the crisp peppermint aroma, and you'll stay toasty warm from the inside out.

16 ounces (475 ml) hot herbal tea (such as peppermint or spearmint)

4 ounces (120 ml) peppermint schnapps

4 ounces (120 ml) apricot schnapps

4 tablespoons (80 g) wildflower honey

Juice of 3 lemons

Make the pot of herbal tea in a teapot. Add the peppermint schnapps and the apricot schnapps, and mix well. Then add the honey and lemon juice (feel free to use a bit more or less, to taste). Serve immediately, or pour into individual flasks and bring them with you into the cold weather for serious warming that'll last for hours. Serves 2 chilly drinkers. ☙

Aquavit with Healing Bitter Herbs and Hot Tea

Caraway seeds, which were traditionally used in topical medicinal prepa-rations, such salves or balms, made their way into the potent Norwegian tipple aquavit, a marvelous caraway- and anise-scented elixir made from potatoes. Taking its name from the Latin phrase aqua vitae, or "water of life," aquavit is also very popular in northern European countries, such as Sweden and Denmark, regions in which below-zero weather is status quo during the winter months. Originally invented in the sixteenth cen-tury as a digestive aid, in the era of the pharmacist and the apothecary, aquavit might have been prepared with other medicinal herbs and sweet spices in addition to caraway, to stave off other cold-weather-induced maladies. It's especially delicious when served on its own alongside platters of smoked fish—or in this healing concoction of aquavit, herb-infused simple syrup, and good old-fashioned hot tea.

1 cup (235 ml) (or more, to taste) hot black tea

2 ounces (60 ml) healing herb simple syrup (see page 155)

3 ounces (90 ml) aquavit

Ground cloves for dusting

Make a pot of strong, hot, black tea, and pour a cup into a large mug. Add the healing herb simple syrup and the aquavit, mixing well after each addition. Dust the top of the drink with the ground cloves. Warm yourself to the bone. Repeat if necessary. ↝

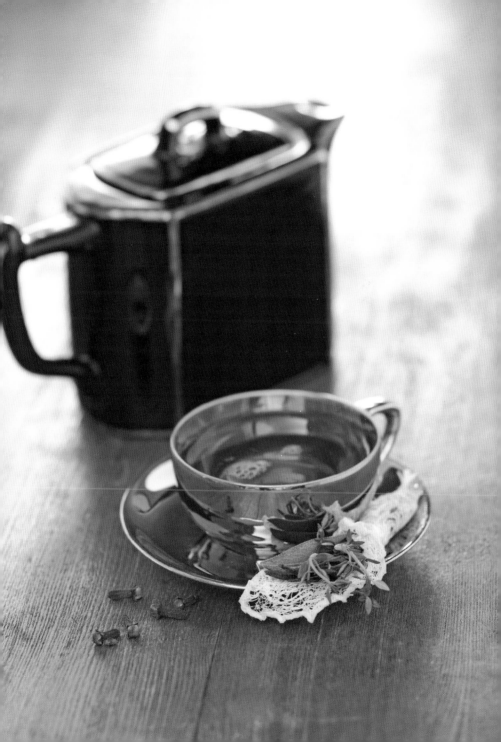

Roasted Beet Borscht with Sour Cream and Vodka

In some of Europe's colder regions, such as eastern Europe and Russia, home cooks add shots of vodka to the roasted-beet-based soup, borscht, then serve it up steaming hot in mugs to help defrost icy fingers. Vodka is often used in these countries as a preservative for dozens of fragile, healing herbs that would otherwise lose their potency. No matter where in the world you are, borscht makes a sturdy, curative meal that's the perfect remedy for damp, frigid weather. (Plus, borscht is a versatile devil: This soup can also be chilled, making for a healthy, refreshing meal in the hot summer months.) Here, it's served up hot in shot glasses with just a nip of vodka for a diminutive yet restorative winter warmer.

3 pounds (1.4 kg) of beets, roasted and puréed (Cut the beets into chunks, and roast in a 350°F [175°C or gas mark 4] oven for 1 hour or until cooked through. Then purée in a blender or food processor until smooth.)

6 cups (1.5 L) strong beef broth (or more to taste, if you prefer a thinner soup)

Freshly grated horseradish, to taste

Vodka

Sour cream for garnish

Add the beef broth to the puréed beets, using a bit more or less broth depending on how you prefer the soup's consistency. Then mix in the horseradish, a little at a time, to taste. Carefully spoon the mixture into individual shot glasses (be careful: the bright-red beet purée stains fabrics). Add 1 medicine-dropperful of vodka to each shot glass. Top each with a small dollop of sour cream. Dig in, and let this Russian elixir perform its healing work upon body and soul. Makes 10 servings, plus leftovers. ❧

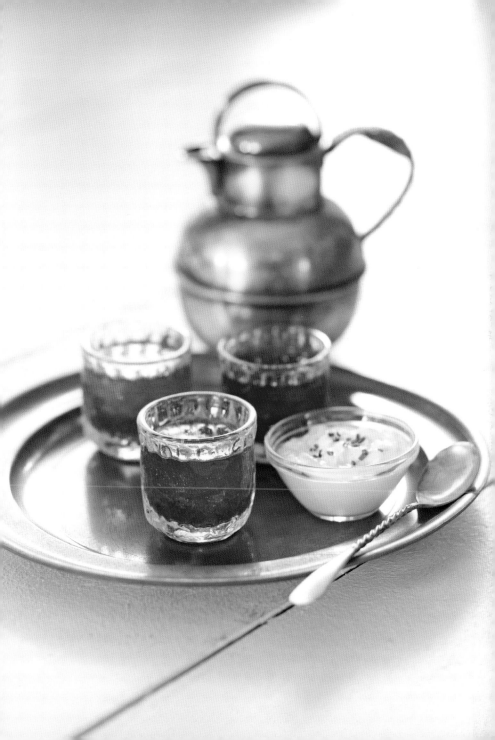

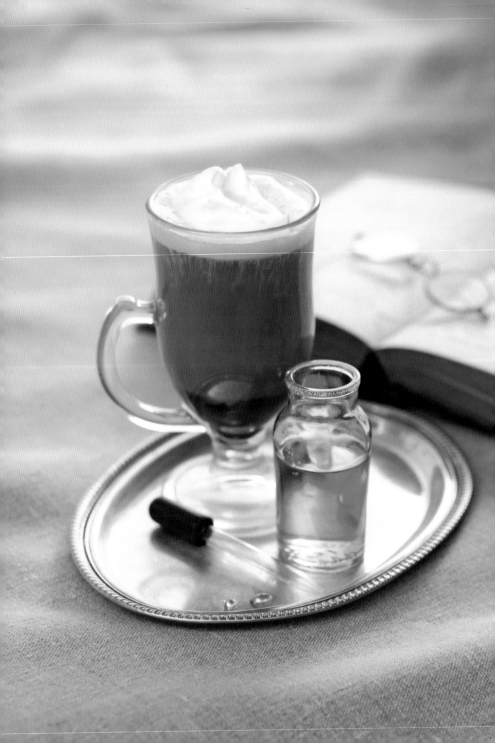

Centerba and Chocolate Chaud

The spicy, potent liqueur Centerba, distilled from over a hundred wild, aromatic (but top-secret) botanicals, hails from northern Italy, a region with a rich history of creating and enjoying herbal Alpine elixirs. Centerba was originally sold in European apothecary shops as a powerful digestive, which was especially useful when the weather was damp and cold. Its alcohol level is nearly 140-proof, making it a most provocative winter warmer for both the head and the belly. How does it taste? When consumed in the form of a hot toddy—that is, combined with boiling water and other ingredients—some say this highly-aromatic elixir is like biting into a hot chili pepper dipped in pinesap. But don't let that put you off. This hot, boozy chill-chaser made with classic hot chocolate— chaud *means "hot" in French—takes the bite off Centerba's acerbic edge.*

3 ounces (90 ml) Centerba

5 to 6 ounces (150 to 175 ml) hot chocolate (combine ¾ cup [175 ml] of whole milk with ¼ cup [60 ml] of heavy cream. Add ¼ pound [115 g] of grated bittersweet chocolate: heat slowly, do not boil, and whisk constantly until smooth.)

Sugar or honey, to taste (optional)

Freshly made whipped cream

Preheat two mugs by filling them with boiling water; discard the water after a few seconds. Add 1½ ounces (45 ml) Centerba to each mug; pour half the hot chocolate over the Centerba in each mug. (Add a little sugar or honey to taste, if necessary.) Spoon the fresh whipped cream over the top—then relax, indulge, and sip until you're thoroughly thawed. Serves 2. ✍

"Corrected" Scotch Broth

One of my favorite winter warmer hails from Scotland, where the Scots "correct" a steaming mug of rich lamb broth with a famous barley-based digestif called—you guessed it—Scotch whisky. Piping-hot Scotch broth is practically a full meal, being packed with lamb, carrots, celery, and onions, and interwoven with lashings of smoky Scotch whisky. (Try to make your own lamb stock for your Scotch broth, since it's so much better than the store-bought stuff.) Like its distant cousin borscht, this fine corrective warms the body, calms the mind, and soothes the spirit— even during the icy winter months when the cold seems to seep into your bones. Can it cure cold-weather maladies? Well, as the Scottish proverb goes, "Whisky may not cure the common cold, but it fails more agreeably than most things."

---

8 ounces (235 ml) lamb stock, either homemade or store-bought, simmered with vegetables of your choice, such as onions, carrots, celery, and potatoes—best simmered in a cast iron pot on a wood-fired stove!

3 ounces (90 ml) very smoky Scotch whisky

Pour the steaming lamb stock with vegetables into a bowl. Add the Scotch whisky, and mix gently. Grab a spoon, and get ready: This curative broth will warm you from the inside out for hours. ❧

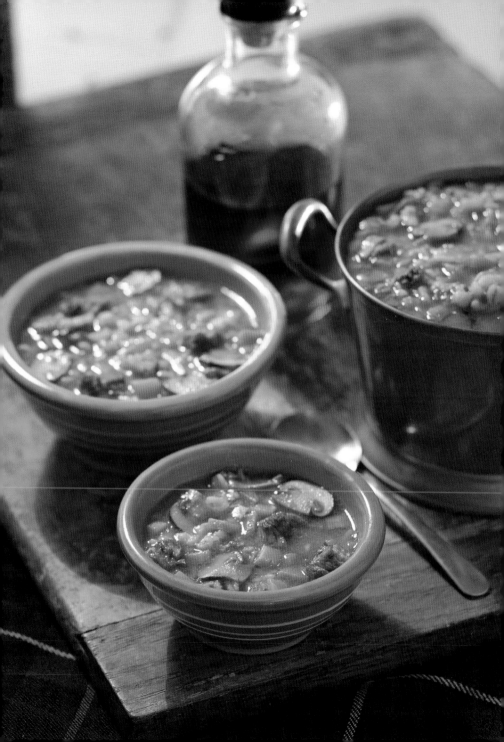

Krupnikas and Hot Tea

Krupnikas, the unique herbal elixir indigenous to Lithuania, can be found in regions of the United States in which Lithuanian immigrants made their homes, such as Cleveland, Ohio, where winters tend to be long and frigid. Eastern Europe boasts a long tradition of using raw honey and potent, distilled alcohol in medicinal, root-based elixirs, and when it comes to counteracting a chill of Arctic proportions, Krupnikas is just what the apothecary ordered. Comprised of herbs, spices, and raw honey combined with alcoholic spirits of nearly 140-proof, Krupnikas can be sipped straight (although I don't recommend it, unless you have an extremely stout constitution!) or enjoyed over ice with soda water and lemon in the summer. In cold weather, though, it's easy to "correct" a cup of hot tea, coffee, or even a hot bowl of thick cabbage soup with a large portion of the healing liqueur.

---

3 ounces (90 ml) Krupnikas

6 ounces (175 ml) hot black tea

Preheat a large mug by filling it with boiling water; discard the water after a few seconds. Add the Krupnikas to the mug, then fill with the hot tea. Mix gently, enjoy a couple deep lungfuls of the fragrant steam, and let the concoction work its warming magic. ❧

Navy Grog

Today, we know how important vitamin C is to a healthy immune system, especially during the winter months when colds and flu run rampant. During the seventeenth and eighteenth centuries, sailors and ship doctors discovered that citrus fruits could combat scurvy, a disease that afflicted many sailors due to the lack of vitamin C in their diets. Soon afterwards, citrus juices and extracts were added to sailors' daily rations of rum and water—a combination called "grog." If a sailor took ill, a hot, restorative tea might have been added to his regimen of rum, citrus juice, and water. Rum—or "kill-devil," as it was called—has been used as a curative for centuries, and the triumvirate of tea, lemon, and rum was said to relieve fevers and stomach maladies. Easy-to-make and satisfying, hot grog is still delicious today—for "medicinal" uses only, of course.

---

10 ounces (285 ml) hot, strong black tea

6 ounces (175 ml) navy-strength (over 90-proof) rum

6 ounces (175 ml) freshly squeezed lemon juice

Prepare the tea in a teapot. Add 3 ounces (90 ml) each of rum and lemon juice to two mugs, then fill the mugs with the hot tea. Administer in piping-hot doses to two tired sailors until rosy-cheeked and refreshed. ⌁

Hot Buttered Rum:
The Sailor's Cure-All

The hot toddy cocktails we know and love today have their roots in the days of yore, when apothecaries might have prescribed them for relief against the aches and pains the Siberian-strength cold weather brings on. Hot toddies are cocktails in which hot or boiling water is added to spirits and other ingredients, and many of these tasty, warming tipples were created to ease cold and flu symptoms. Ships' doctors of yesteryear may have delivered doses of this classic hot buttered rum to sailors to relieve aching bones and flagging spirits. Four magic ingredients—hot tea, sugar, butter, and rum—connect every sailor who's ever had to head face-first into a full gale while out at sea. Today, this curative is a treat that goes down smoothly after a long day of skiing, hiking, or just sitting by the fire.

Hot black tea

6 ounces (175 ml) rum

Dark brown sugar to taste

2 teaspoons butter (9 g or about 2 acorn-sized lumps)

Freshly grated nutmeg

Prepare a pot of strong black tea. While the tea is steeping, preheat mugs by filling them with boiling water; discard the water after a few seconds.

Add 3 ounces (90 ml) of rum to each mug. Fill each mug with tea and mix gently.

Sweeten to taste with dark brown sugar. Add a acorn-sized lump of butter to each mug, and dust each drink with fresh nutmeg. Anchors aweigh! Serves 2. ⌖

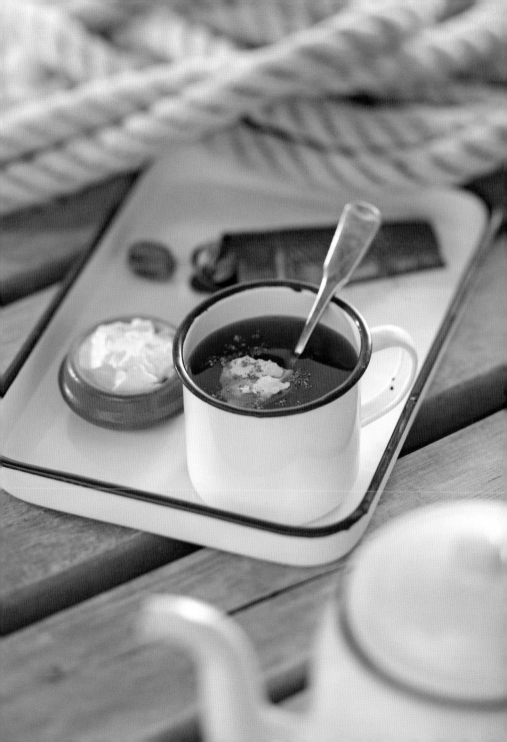

Ginger-Lime Shrubb Cocktail

Okay, so the Ginger-Lime Shrubb Cocktail isn't a hot drink, but it'll warm the cockles of your heart nonetheless. Shrubb cocktails are derived from historic maritime cocktail ingredients that include vinegar for the preservation of easily spoiled—and valuable—citrus fruits. Without preservatives, citrus fruits would have quickly rotted under the hot sun. In traditional Shrubb cocktails, lime and ginger supplement honey, vinegar, and cider, packing powerful health benefits. They take their inspiration from the concentrated citrus syrups once used to stave off tropical diseases that plagued seafarers, such as scurvy. The intense flavors of lime and ginger can act as an antidote to seasickness on their own, but they're especially delicious alongside rum and hydrating, refreshing seltzer water—particularly soothing when fighting a body-ravaging cold.

3 ounces (90 ml) Rhum Agricole

3 to 4 tablespoons (45 to 60 ml) ginger–lime Shrubb syrup (See page 156)

Seltzer water

Several dashes of Angostura bitters

Ice

Toss a handful of ice cubes into a short rocks glass. Add the Rhum Agricole and stir in the ginger-lime Shrubb syrup. Top with the seltzer water and a dash or two of stomach-healing Angostura bitters, to taste. Sip slowly, letting the bracing ginger-lime combination nurse you back to health. ⌁

3 Hot-Weather Refreshers ✣

Drinks to Cool the Fevered Brow

he mere mention of the word summer conjures up heavenly visions: long days spent at the beach, surrounded by the scents of salt water and sun-cream; slices of watermelon the size of your head; fireflies glowing at dusk; and barbeques with friends that stretch late into the night. But when the temperature soars above ninety—or even into the triple digits— the heat can be pretty hard to bear. Those dog days of summer make us long for a cool spell; so we shut out the heat, hunker down under the AC, and dream of all things arctic.

Quit dreaming and start pouring! The fact is hot climates require powerful preparations for cooling the body from the inside out. Sure, medicinal, steamy-hot toddies are as effective—and delicious—in summer as they are in winter, but apothecaries knew that the best way to relieve their patients of what ailed them during the summer months was to prescribe curatives that would refresh as well as heal. Rejuvenating alcoholic drinks, such as tonics, flips, fizzes, and punches all have powerful healing properties when combined with herbs, spices, citrus fruits, and even fresh, garden-grown vegetables. (Traditionally, pharmacists would have used alcohol as a preservative, keeping delicate herbs and spices from being spoiled, even in sweltering heat.) Of course, it's important to drink plenty of plain water year-round to stay healthy, but fresh citrus juices used in hot-weather cocktails, such as orange, lemon, and lime, also offer a hit of hydration in addition to vitamin C. Drinks that call for fizzy water, such as club soda or seltzer, help you feel cooler a bit quicker thanks to those refreshing little bubbles, and can help restore appetites that wilt in the summer sun.

"Fruits and vegetables from your own garden pack powerful healing properties, too—and it'd be a crime not to use them in summer drinks when they're so abundant this time of year."

Using exotic spices and flavorful ingredients, such as hot chiles, in cocktails can help bring down body temperature and aid healing. When we eat spicy foods such as chiles, we tend to sweat, which creates moisture on the surface of the skin. When the wind blows across damp skin, you feel cooler immediately. That's why a *Roasted Tomato and Chile Bloody Mary* enjoyed in the heat of the sun is so effective against overheating: It literally cools you from the inside out. Anise, a key ingredient in the French liqueur Pernod and the Turkish liqueur raki, the key ingredient in *Almond Pastis*, is renowned as a relaxant for both body and mind, and as a cure for all manner of digestive disorders. It's no accident that it's often enjoyed before or after meals—it soothes the belly and calms the brain. Also, fresh coconuts, which take center stage in the *Coconut Cooler*, carry precious potassium in the fragrant water within them—perhaps that explains why the piña colada is such a popular beach-weather tipple.

But cooling cocktails aren't always about exotic flavors. Fruits and vegetables from your own garden pack powerful healing properties, too—and it'd be a crime not to use them in summer drinks when they're so abundant this time of year. Humble, tart rhubarb, which usually gets the spotlight only in desserts, such as pies, tarts, and cobblers, has actually been used in healing for more than 200 years, and it's delicious in drinks such as the *Rhubarb Fizz with Charred Strawberries*. And, if you ask me, the tomato is one of the most misunderstood of the garden-to-glass ingredients—it's incredibly effective in healing and cooling, since it's both hydrating and loaded with the antioxidant lycopene, so there's no reason to say no to a Bloody Mary. (The best part? They're so flavorful that even the virgin variety doesn't skimp on taste.)

Finally, you don't have to take your medicine on your own: These hot-weather tipples are real people-pleasers. If you've invited a swarm of thirsty friends for a barbeque, whip up some citrusy *Rum Punch for a Crowd*, an easy-to-make combo of freshly squeezed juices, rum, and aromatic bitters served up over ice. Or toss off a few batches of the *Nix Besser Cocktail*, a veritable summer salad of roasted peaches, Thai basil, and chiles mixed with rum and rye whiskey.

Sweltering weather can make even the most vivacious folks flag a bit, but don't slink indoors to hide from the heat—let these chilled-out cocktails inspired by the apothecary help you embrace it.

Note for the Reader:

All recipes make a single serving, unless otherwise indicated.
All herbs are fresh, unless otherwise indicated.

Rocks from the Tropics

Instead of using plain ice cubes in your refreshers, why not try freezing some coconut water in a solution of 40 percent coconut water to 60 percent filtered water? What you will find is a frozen method of adding flavor to your drinks without adding too much extra volume to the final product. Plus, as the ice melts into the liquor, the flavor of your drink will change and become more concentrated and elegant.

Roasted Tomato and Chili Bloody Mary

One of the best things about summertime is its abundance of fresh fruit and vegetables: Gardens and farmers' markets overflow with juicy melons, succulent strawberries, delicate lettuces, and firm, deep-red tomatoes. It's the perfect time to cool down with this spicy twist on the classic Bloody Mary, which puts those magnificent tomatoes to good use by popping them into the oven. (Trust me, the rich flavor of roasted tomatoes really makes it worth turning on the oven, even in sizzling heat.) Tomatoes are chock full of disease-fighting antioxidants, and lemon juice packs a healthy wallop of vitamin C, while celery seeds are said to possess anti-inflammatory properties. Plus, this spunky version of the Bloody Mary is just as delicious sans the vodka.

6 ounces (175 ml) good-quality vodka

6 ounces (175 ml) roasted tomato purée (see page 157)

3 ounces (90 ml) lemon juice

2 tablespoons (30 ml) hot chili sauce (a sweet-and-spicy one works best, such as Vietnamese sriracha)

Ice cubes

Dash of celery salt

Combine all the ingredients except the celery salt in a large glass, and mix gently (with a celery stick, perhaps?). Just before serving, sprinkle the celery salt over the top of the drink. Garnish with a lemon wedge. Find a spot in the shade, sip slowly, and cool down from the inside out. Serves 2. ⟋

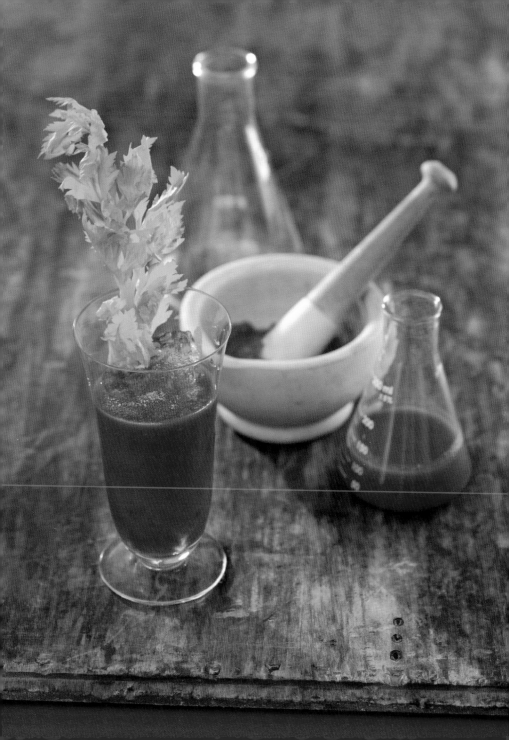

Rhubarb and Strawberry Swizzle

Rhubarb has been prescribed as a curative for hundreds of years. That's because it's a good source of vitamin C and potassium—and, some say, is even an aphrodisiac. The strawberry-rhubarb combo is also delicious in cooling cocktails: It mixes marvelously with rum, particularly Rhum Agricole, a type of rum distilled from sugar cane in the West Indian island of Martinique. There, "kill-devil" was used in traditional curatives—but don't worry, if you can't find Rhum Agricole, any good quality spiced rum will do. The rock candy swizzle stick adds just the right amount of sweetness to the mix, while the effervescence of club soda gives wilting spirits a lift.

3 tablespoons (45 ml) strawberry-rhubarb compote (Roughly chop four stalks of rhubarb. In a medium saucepan, combine one pint [290 g] of strawberries and the rhubarb, and place over medium heat until softened. Using a food processor or mortar and pestle, purée the mixture until it becomes a thick liquid. Set aside to cool.)

6 ounces (175 ml) Rhum Agricole (or Cachaca rum, if you can't find it)

1 rock candy swizzle stick

12 ounces (355 ml) club soda

Ice cubes

Add the strawberry and rhubarb mixture, rum, and ice to a glass beaker, and mix well with the swizzle stick. (The faster you swizzle, the better! Moving the swizzle stick quickly ensures that the liquids and solids in the drink are thoroughly combined.) Strain the mixture into two coupé glasses, top with club soda, and use the swizzle stick as garnish, if desired. Then kick back and let the tart, refreshing fizz chill you out. Serves 2. ↷

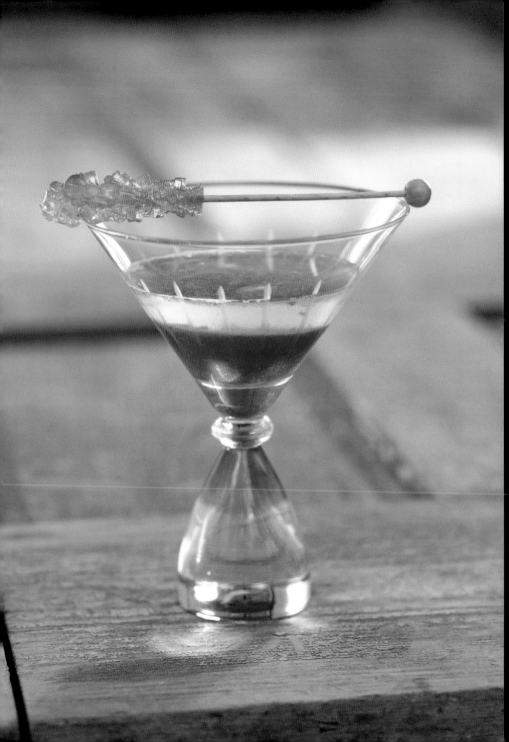

Branca Menta and Cola

If a Cuba Libre is your usual warm-weather tipple, skip the rum for once, and kick things up a notch with a Branca Menta and Cola. Since time immemorial, potent herbal digestifs such as Branca Menta have been mixed with cool water, ice, and sugar to relieve tired, overheated bodies. Like its Italian cousin, Fernet Branca, it's an aromatic, herbal liqueur that contains over forty (top-secret!) herbs, plus an extra dose of menthol and peppermint, both of which cool down the body and mellow out the mind. It also contains anise, which as any apothecary worth his salt would tell you, adds a crisp licorice flavor to the mix and encourages relaxation. This bracing cocktail rounds out the Menta with a hit of cola, which takes the bitter edge off the liqueur's remedial botanicals.

3 ounces (90 ml) Branca Menta

6 ounces (175 ml) cane sugar cola (or regular cola)

Ice cubes

Pack a tall glass with ice cubes. Pour the Branca Menta over the ice—you'll feel revitalized after just a whiff of its bracing scent. Add the cola slowly, and sip your way to relief. ⟿

Orange Zest Oasis

Anise has been used in curatives at least since the Middle Ages. It's often taken as a digestif after meals (and therefore pops up in desserts and sweet treats around the world—think black jelly beans). But it's also said to calm and cool hot, parched bodies from the inside out. During long spells of hot, steamy weather, pharmacists of old may have prepared tonics that offered relief from scorching days and sultry nights. They might have combined anise and other herbs with hot peppers—which would make patients sweat, helping them feel cooler fast—and preserve them in a heavy dose of high-proof alcohol. This sweet-and-bitter cocktail takes its inspiration from just such a combination (minus the hot peppers, of course). Here, muddled oranges bathed in dry sake offset the fragrant anisette.

2 orange slices, cut into quarters

½ tablespoon (7 ml) root tea syrup (see page 155)

¼ ounce (7 ml) anisette

3 ounces (90 ml) dry sake

4 drops Thai bitters

1 egg white

Orange zest twist

Put the orange slices in the bottom of a Boston shaker, and muddle with a cocktail stick or the long end of a wooden spoon. Then add the remaining ingredients, one at a time. Shake them well for thirty seconds. Strain the frothy mixture into a coupé glass. Garnish with a flamed orange zest twist (pinch the zest firmly and hold it behind a lit match to release the citrusy oils). It's the perfect way to beat the heat. ➤

Rum Punch for a Crowd

Citrus-laden rum punch was an early—and effective—curative for the evils of heat waves. In Caribbean areas, such as Martinique or Haiti, both of which bear influences of French culture and its healing techniques, an apothecary would traditionally prescribe rum-based potions containing locally gathered herbs and spices, plus lashings of aromatic bitters. These healing potions would help soothe anyone who was suffering from the weather—even in the midst of the most oppressive heat and humidity. These medicinal "cocktails" evolved into rum punches, which are still made and enjoyed today. Made with fresh citrus juices and a healthy dose of light rum over ice and a whack of seltzer water, a bowl of punch is a delightful way to refresh and relax a crowd of thirsty revelers.

---

1 bottle (750 ml) of rum

1 bottle (750 ml) of overproof (160–190-proof) rum

1 quart (950 ml) each of citrus juice (such as orange, grapefruit, lemon, lime— freshly-squeezed is best)

1 bottle (750 ml) club soda

1 to 2 tablespoons (15 to 30 ml), Angostura bitters

Ice cubes

Fill a large punch bowl half full with ice. Pour the rum over the ice, adding the fruit juices one at a time, and mix well with a wooden spoon—then replace the spoon with a ladle so your parched guests can serve themselves. Serves at least 10 to 15 thirsty partygoers. ↷

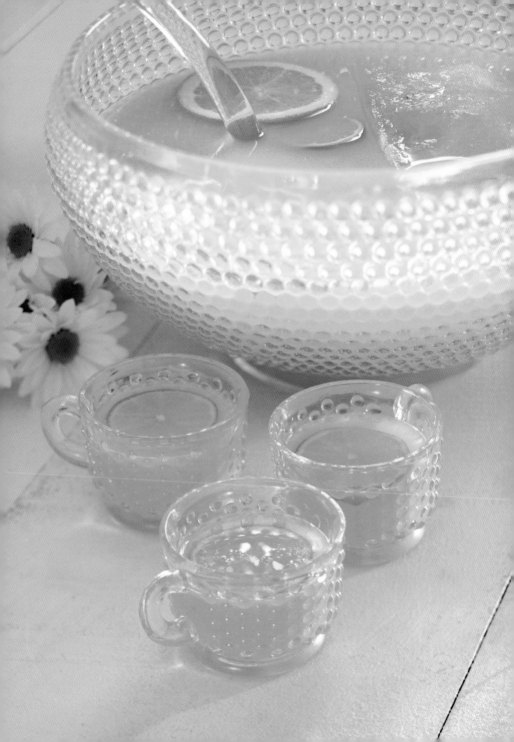

Rhubarb Fizz with Charred Strawberries

Fizzes are delicious, revitalizing preparations that suspend healing botanicals, liquors, and/or juices in seltzer water, and the Rhubarb Fizz is a famous—or infamous—example. Rhubarb has been used in traditional Chinese medicine for thousands of years, and it has been used in the United States since at least the eighteenth century as a remedy for digestive disorders. This curative fizz adds charred strawberries to citrusy, spicy, organic rhubarb liqueur, and it's a marriage made in heaven. Add some botanical gin, the effervescence of seltzer water, and plenty of crushed ice, and you've got a cooling cocktail that restores both overheated bodies and flagging spirits.

¼ cup (40 g) charred strawberries (sear strawberries in a cast-iron pan over very high heat, then set aside until cool)

3 ounces (90 ml) 80-proof rhubarb tea liqueur (preferably organic)

1 ounce (30 ml) botanical gin

Ice cubes

1 ounce (30 ml) simple syrup (see page 155)

Seltzer water

Crushed ice

Add about 2 tablespoons (30 g) of the charred strawberries and the simple syrup to a Boston shaker. Muddle them until they make a fragrant pulp. Then add the rhubarb tea liqueur and the botanical gin, and pile the crushed ice over the liquors and strawberries until the shaker is three-quarters full. Shake well for twenty seconds, scoop some of the crushed ice into a coupé glass (its texture will have become slushy), strain the mixture over the ice, and top with seltzer water. Prepare to be healed! ↝

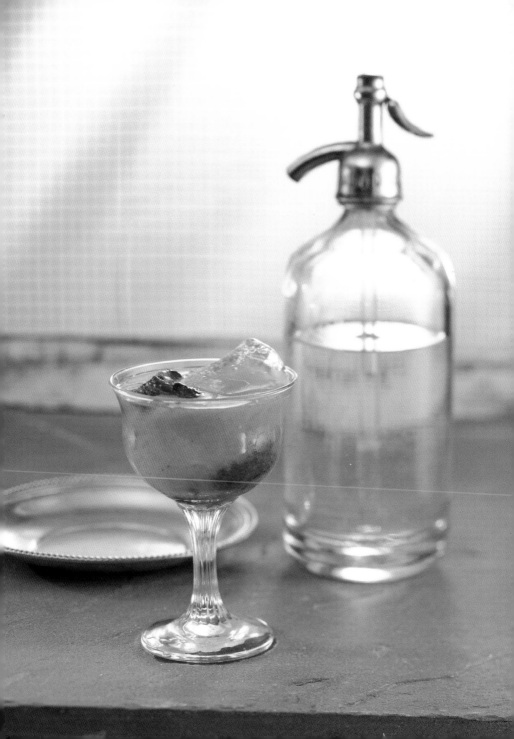

Almond Pastis

Pastis is one of the most popular drinks in France, especially in the nation's southern and southwestern regions, where scorching heat can accompany the summer months. The French, undisputed masters of all things gastronomic, rely on this simple cocktail of aniseed-flavored liqueur diluted with water and served over ice to keep that stifling heat at bay. It can be enjoyed as an aperitif, digestif, or even on its own during those long, warm afternoons. Here, an infusion of orgeat—that is, almond-flavored—syrup acts as a delicious foil to the liqueur's bitter edge. If you like, you can substitute Turkish raki for the Pernod—both work equally well.

3 ounces (90 ml) French
Pernod or Turkish raki

2 ounces (60 ml) orgeat
syrup

6 ounces (175 ml) cool water

Ice cubes

Add a handful of ice cubes to a 12-ounce (355 ml) glass. Add the Pernod or raki, followed by the orgeat syrup. Pour the cool water over the liqueur and syrup, and mix gently. It's just what the apothecary ordered to restore wilting appetites before a meal—especially alongside hors d'oeuvres or a Turkish mezze platter of olives, cheeses, dips, and fresh fruits and vegetables. ➙

Pompier Cocktail

Vermouth served chilled over ice is another famous warm-weather refresher. Vermouth comes in two forms: sweet or dry, and each is delicious when served on its own over ice or with the addition of other liquors such as rye whiskey or Scotch. Historically, pharmacists may have prescribed vermouth as a remedy for afflictions that were exacerbated by hot weather, including intestinal disorders and gout. Created by my fellow cocktail scribe, Gary Regan, this cocktail was based on the Pompier Highball that's detailed in the fabulous Gentleman's Companion: An Exotic Drinking Book *by Charles Baker, Jr., published in 1946. It features a dash of vitamin-laden citrus and a tot of gin to make the medicine go down, as they say, "with a grin of sin on your face." It's fairly low in alcohol, so add a bit more gin to it, if you like, but avoid using more than one ounce (30 ml), since it's really the herbs in the vermouth that make this drink a curative treat.*

2.5 ounces (75 ml) dry vermouth

½ ounce (15 ml) gin

¼ ounce (7 ml) crème de cassis

Lemon twist

Ice

Fill a Boston shaker three-quarters full with ice. Add the liquid ingredients one at a time, stir gently, and strain into a chilled cocktail glass. Garnish with the lemon twist. Take one each time the temperature hits ninety!

Coconut Cooler

In the Caribbean islands, pharmacists of days gone by might have been called on to help patients counter the effects of too much sun. Their solution was probably a simple one, relying on potassium-packed coconut water for hydration and local rum to ease the sufferer's body and mind. Pharmacists may have packed their coconuts in ice overnight to ensure that the coconut water—the nutrient-dense, milky liquid inside the fruit—was well-chilled before punching holes in them to pour a healthy dose of rum inside. Since coconut water has more potassium than two bananas, it's a speedy way to replenish much-needed nutrients in the midst of mind-boggling heat. And the best part is, there's no glass to wash afterwards.

One large coconut, chilled

6 ounces (175 ml) Rhum Agricole

Chill the coconut by keeping it on ice overnight, or by storing it in the refrigerator. Using a drill, puncture three holes into the coconut (but don't discard the precious water inside!). In the islands, a machete is often used to punch holes into coconuts. Some people who use machetes are missing their fingertips. I'm not one of them.

Add the Rhum Agricole through one of the holes, using a funnel if necessary. Stick a straw into each of the holes, and sip the contents while cheek-to-cheek with a close friend. Serves 2. ↷

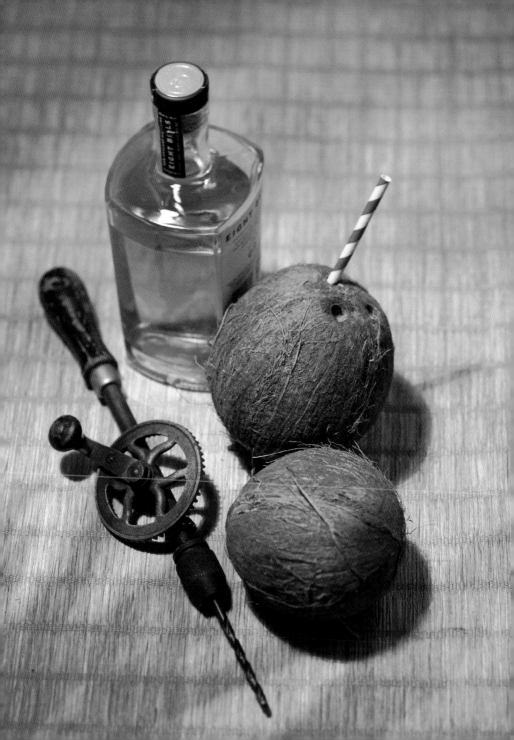

Nix Besser Cocktail

Nix besser means "none better" in Amish, and this cocktail lives up to its name. Here, fresh, roasted peaches partner with the summery flavors of chiles, simple syrup, and Thai basil—and they make a run for bibulous infamy when combined with rye whiskey and freshly squeezed-citrus juices. Apothecaries might have recommended this cocktail because it is said to help heal a number of maladies, including heatstroke—plus, the peach has been used in traditional Chinese medicine for centuries to improve circulation and to relieve the symptoms of allergies.

2 tablespoons (30 ml) of roasted peaches (slice about a pound [455 g] of fresh peaches into chunks, then roast for about 25 minutes at 400°F [200°C or gas mark 6], or until caramelized and soft. Set aside to cool. Purée in a food processor until they become a soft pulp)

4 ounces (120 ml) rye whiskey

3 ounces (90 ml) spiced rum

4 tablespoons (60 ml) Royal Rose Simple Syrup with Chilies

3 ounces (90 ml) freshly squeezed lime juice

3 ounces (90 ml) freshly squeezed orange juice

Several Thai basil leaves, sliced

2 tablespoons (30 ml) aromatic bitters

Ice cubes

Put all of the ingredients except the bitters and ice cubes into a tall mixing glass. Stir gently—but whatever you do, don't shake! Add the bitters to the mixture. Put four ice cubes into two Collins glasses. Divide the mixture between the two glasses, and you'll see how this cocktail got its name: There really is nothing better for keeping the heat at bay. ⟩

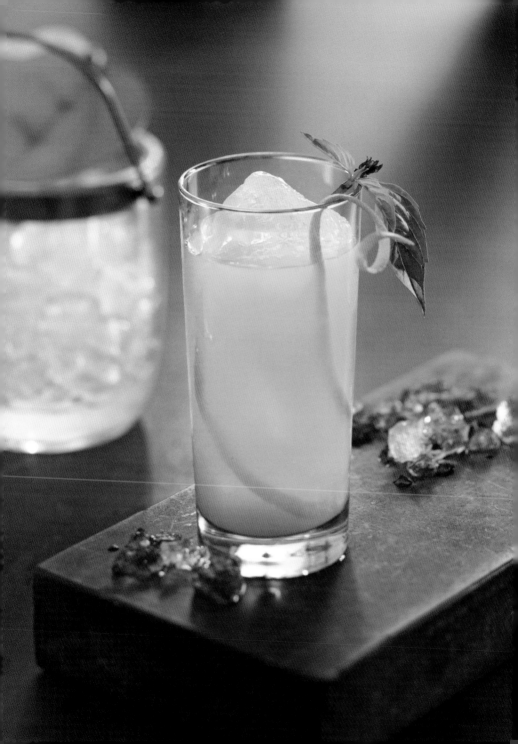

4 Restoratives

Tasted-And-True Hangover Cures from the Apothecary

angover: The very word is enough to fill any committed drinker's heart with fear. Most of the time it's easy to say no to another neat whiskey or to turn your back on that umpteenth toddy, but every once in a while, everyone ends up enjoying themselves a bit too much on an evening out. The next morning, all the classic symptoms appear: a throbbing head, a belly in turmoil, eyelids that make a scratching noise when you blink, and exhaustion so profound that you utter those five dreaded words: I'm never drinking again. Ever.

Never fear: Hangovers are nothing new, as any pharmacist of old could tell you. Prescriptive cures for the aftereffects of booze abounded in days of yore, since food was much heavier, as a rule, and more of it was consumed during meals. *Bon vivants* of the past would have been more likely to consume many different kinds of liquors at a single sitting, creating a veritable stew of distemper for the belly and the head. Plus, kitchen hygiene, both at home and in restaurants, may not have been as strictly observed as it is today. So, it's no surprise that the imbiber might need a bit of help waking up the morning after a particularly vigorous night of eating and drinking (followed by more eating and drinking). Back in the day, at a Bacchanalian event called a Beefsteak, men gathered together for an all-you-can-eat beef-, beer-, and liquor-fest. Donning white aprons to catch splatterings of grease and spirits, partygoers got gluttonous—and kept going long into the night. The aftermath the next morning required seriously strong medicine—in the form of tasty, restorative cocktails.

Restoratives often combine herbs, spices, and citrus fruits to perk up the senses and lighten the heart after a late night. After all, a restorative should perk up your pulse and make you feel wide-awake—whether that's in the morning or evening is up to you! Historically, restoratives were powerful incorporations of spices, ranging in flavors from bitter to sweet. During the Paris Exposition of 1878, a stomach-turning combination of raw egg yolks mixed with Worcestershire sauce, Tabasco sauce, salt, and pepper became famous as a cure for the most explosive hangovers: later, the addition of overproof vodka and tomato juice made the foul mixture more palatable, and literally scared the pain right out of the sufferer's head. It worked, but it certainly wasn't for the faint of heart.

Alternatively, after a night of overindulgence, a dulled palate might be revived by the addition of lemon or lime juice to a cocktail, or by flaming the zest, or peel, of a citrus fruit before adding it to a drink—it's especially aromatic (and healing). Here's how: Hold a slice of citrus peel just behind a lit match, pinch it to release its natural oils, and then direct the oily spray into your glass, and enjoy the heady scents of warm citrus and toasty caramel. Stone fruits, such as plums and peaches, can be puréed or macerated with alcohol to offer healing relief for sore heads and stomach maladies of all kinds. Historically, a pharmacist might have added aromatic flower water to his restorative potions, since its sumptuous citrus flavors were known to relax the regretful drinker and lighten his aching spirits. (In fact, modern-day versions of botanical gin sometimes include orange flower water for these very reasons.) Other equally effective restoratives take the form of a milk punch: Drenched in both heavy cream and milk, these stomach-coating elixirs rescue sufferers from the throes of even the most wicked hangovers. Most importantly, though, any cocktail meant to lift the spirit after a difficult night out on the town should also be enticing both to the nose and the eyes, and it never hurts to serve restorative cocktails in a tall glass with plenty of ice.

"Extract of milk thistle has been used to heal vehement hangovers for centuries, due to its natural liver-healing qualities."

Whatever your poison, there's a cure to be found for it. Pharmacists of old often pre-scribed tonics including lighter spirits, such as gin, white rum, or vodka to heal debili-tating hangovers—or, they may have suggested the simple combination of homemade, healing bitters and salted soda water, served over ice in a tall glass. It's a cure that's still delicious—and effective—today. The judicious use of Angostura or Peychaud's bitters, along with freshly drawn seltzer water, is always a pleasure to drink, especially if an angry stomach ailment rears its ugly head. Extract of milk thistle has been used to heal vehement hangovers for centuries, due to its natural liver-healing qualities. An extra shot of the Italian herbal liqueur Fernet Branca is still hailed as a quick, effective remedy for sore heads and bellies. In this chapter, you'll find more recipes that are sure to cure—from the wonderfully effervescent *Thai Basil Fizz*, to the cooling *Painkiller Prescriptive*, a rum-based cocktail with a tropical edge. Or, if you feel like the undead after an evening of debauchery, let the cognac-heavy *Corpse Reviver* bring you back to the land of the living. Just what the pharmacist ordered!

Note for the Reader:

All recipes make a single serving, unless otherwise indicated.
All herbs are fresh, unless otherwise indicated.

Cocktail Whisperer's Recommendation

Drink a tall glass of white rum with freshly squeezed sweet citrus juices, like grapefruit and orange. Add a splash of seltzer and some aromatic bitters like Angostura for a refreshing, quick pick-me-up.

Fernet Branca Shots

Fernet Branca has been used as a powerful hangover remedy for generations. Since its invention in nineteenth-century Italy, Fernet's qualities as a soothing digestif after a large meal have spread far and wide. Made with dozens of herbs from all over the world, the recipe for Fernet Branca is top-secret, but we do know it has a great history as a fixer-upper for flagging spirits: A few ice-cold shots of Fernet are known to vanquish pesky hangovers nearly immediately. (Then again, the 80-proof spirits may also have something to do with it.) Either way, a quick dose of Fernet Branca the morning (or afternoon) after will leave you wide-awake and ready to take on a new day—hangover-free.

1 ounce (30 ml) Fernet Branca

Dash of ginger beer

Simply add one shot of Fernet Branca to a short glass, then top with ginger beer or ginger ale. (Don't add ice.) Pay no attention to your aching head: Lift your glass, down the contents, and repeat if necessary. Salut!

Sambuca Twist

*One of my favorite restorative cocktails, this tipple features Sambuca,
which can act as a powerful wake-me-up for a stressed-out stomach.
The freshly squeezed grapefruit juice adds a much-needed dose of
vitamin C, while the citrusy, singed orange peel and the licorice-flavored
Sambuca combine to reanimate the spirits of even the most zealous
drinker. Even if you're not usually a fan of the liqueur's distinctive
aniseed scent and taste, you'll be amazed at how healing and
refreshing the Sambuca Twist is after a hard night out on the tiles.*

4 ounces (120 ml) botanical gin

1 ounce (30 ml) Sambuca

3 ounces (90 ml) freshly squeezed grapefruit juice

Slice of fresh orange peel

Several shakes of aromatic bitters, such as Peychaud's

Grapefruit zest twist

Ice

Add the gin, Sambuca, and grapefruit juice to a Boston shaker. Shake vigorously for fifteen seconds. Add a handful of ice cubes to a Collins glass, and strain the mixture over the ice. Singe a slice of fresh orange peel, pinching it firmly just behind the match to release its natural citrus oils, and then add it to the glass. Finally, shake the bitters into the drink, and garnish with the grapefruit zest twist. Your stomach will thank you after just a few sips. ➷

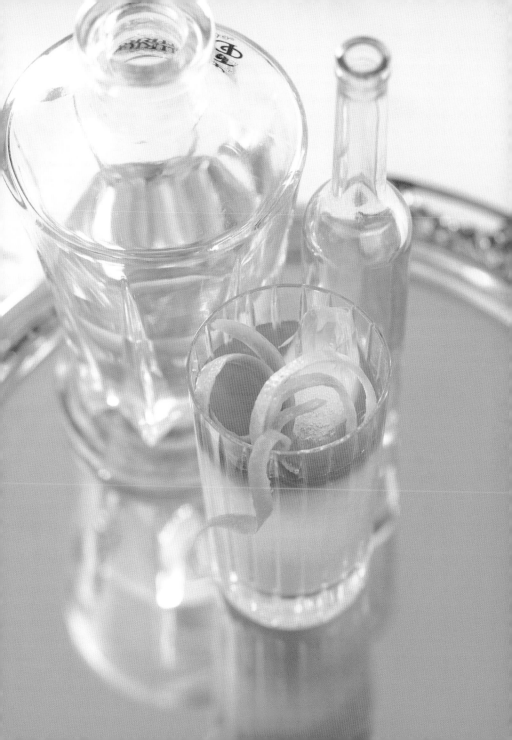

Corpse Reviver

Corpse Revivers were designed for a truly horrible hangover—the kind that won't let you lift your head off the pillow. True to its name, a Corpse Reviver is meant to re-animate the dead—or, at least, the vividly hung over. This potent combination of cognac, gin, apple brandy, and vermouth mixed with falernum—a liqueur sporting a heady mixture of Caribbean flavors, such as almond, ginger, cloves, vanilla, and lime— takes the sting out of even the most heinous of hangovers. Falernum gets its name from an ancient Roman wine called falernian, which, legend has it, was so high in alcohol it could be set on fire. Here, a hearty dose of cognac soothes the pain of the night before, while the fragrant falernum rejuvenates all five aching senses.

---

3 ounces (90 ml) cognac

2 ounces (60 ml) calvados

1 ounce (30 ml) gin

1 ounce (30 ml) sweet vermouth

1 ounce (30 ml) falernum

Ice

Fill a Boston shaker three-quarters full with ice. Gently pour the cognac, calvados, gin, vermouth, and falernum over the ice, and shake briskly for thirty seconds.

Toss a few ice cubes into a short rocks glass. Strain the mixture into the glass, sit back, and slowly sip that hangover away.

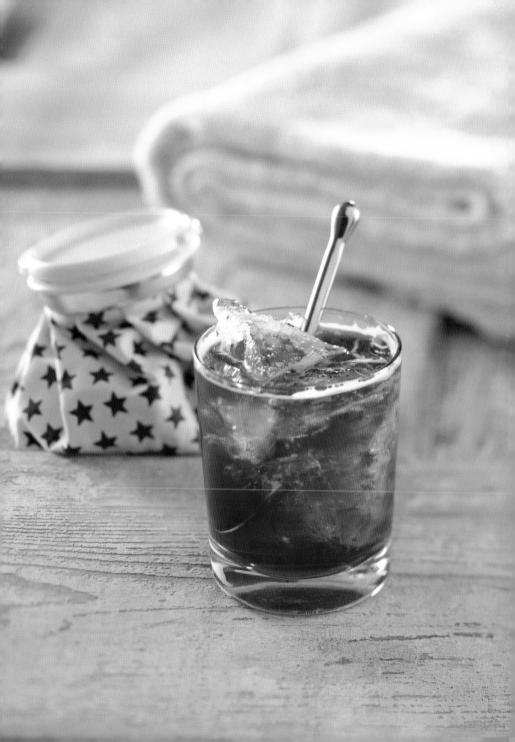

Ramos Gin Fizz Cocktail

Like the Corpse Reviver, this deliciously fizzy cocktail is effective against the most brutal hangovers. Designed to heal the adverse effects of late nights without doing damage to sensitive stomachs, it combines fragrant orange flower water with gin, frothed egg white, half-and-half, sugar, milk, lemon juice, and lots of fizzy soda water. Then it's shaken for several minutes to "cook" the egg whites and make for a softly fizzy cocktail that is a powerful emulsifier for maladies of the belly and your aching head (orange flower water has been known to ease headaches and calm jazzy nerves). The creamy quality of the egg whites and the half-and-half soothe the belly in ways totally unappreciated until a hangover actually occurs. If you're really feeling rough, get someone else to shake the cocktail for you; remember, no sudden movements.

3 ounces (90 ml) gin

3 drops orange flower water

3 egg whites

½ teaspoon bar sugar (or powdered sugar)

1 ounce (30 ml) lemon juice

¼ teaspoon vanilla extract

2 ounces (60 ml) club soda

Dash of salt

2 ounces (60 ml) half-and-half

1 ounce (30 ml) whole milk

Fill a Boston shaker three-quarters full of ice. One at a time, add all the ingredients to it, and mix well.

Shake well for at least two minutes. (Legend has it that real connoisseurs shake their Ramos Ginn Fizzes for upwards of ten minutes!) You'll be thirsty long before that: When your arm gets tired, strain the mixture into a large glass, and prepare to be healed. ⚘

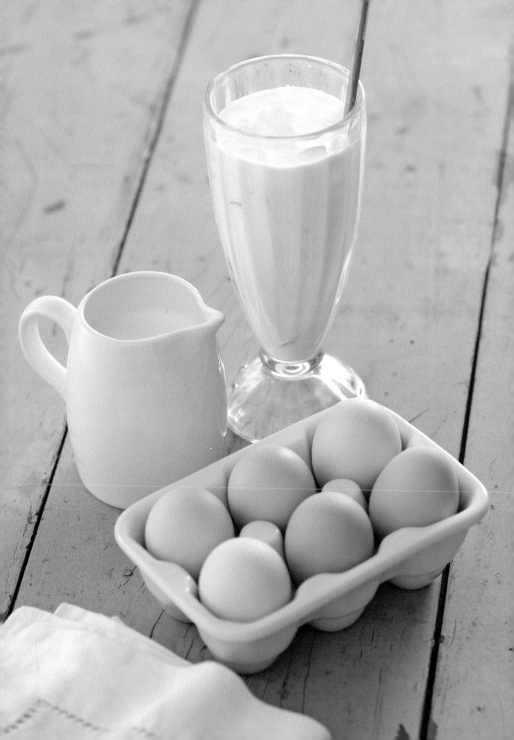

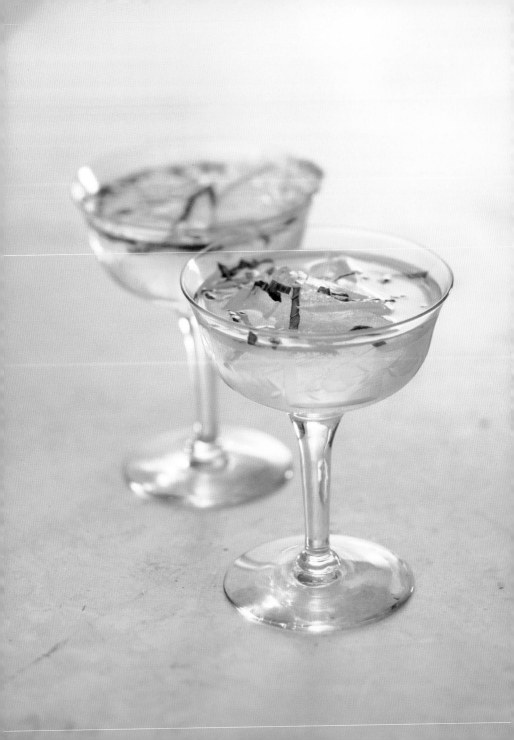

Thai Basil Fizz

Basil: It's not just for pesto anymore. Basil, with its bracing, peppery taste, is often used in curatives. It was said to mitigate the symptoms of malaria, and was made into a liniment to soothe sunburns. Basil was also used as a nerve tonic against stress and anxiety, and it is even said to promote longevity. One variety of the herb, called holy basil or Thai basil, is used as an ingredient alongside other green herbs in both absinthe and green chartreuse, due to its antiseptic and antibacterial qualities. (In fact, the striking green color of absinthe and chartreuse may pay homage to basil's brilliant green hue.) Thai basil can be very effective when it comes to healing a sour stomach: Try a Thai Basil Fizz if you spent last night indulging in spicy food washed down by one too many cocktails.

---

1 sprig holy basil (or regular basil), finely chopped

2 ounces (60 ml) botanical gin

¼ ounce (7 ml) absinthe

3 to 4 shakes of Peychaud's bitters

2 to 3 ounces (60 to 90 ml) ginger beer

Lemon zest twist

Ice

Toss the chopped basil into a Boston shaker. (Be sure to lean over the shaker for a restorative whiff of its crisp, spicy scent!) Add the gin and absinthe, and fill the shaker three-quarters full of ice. Sprinkle the bitters into the mix, then shake for twenty seconds, strain into a coupé glass, and top with the ginger beer. Garnish with the lemon zest twist. The heady combination of basil, ginger, and lemon is sure to brush the cobwebs away.

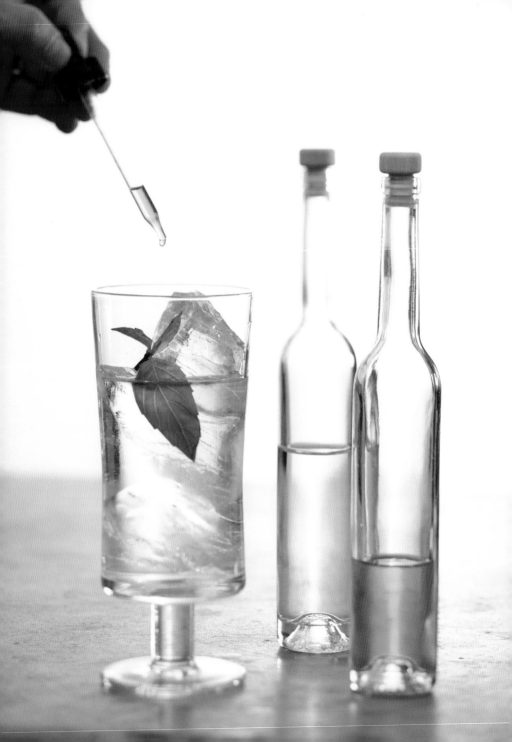

Gin and Coconut Ice with Seltzer

Some hangover remedies act as a welcome slap in the face for tired taste buds and jolt the senses back to life with a bang. If your body and mind feel a bit on the delicate side, though, you crave a tipple that'll ease you back to the land of the living as painlessly as possible. This delicious tonic takes the edge off an ornery stomach in a gentle way, combining gin, fizzy seltzer, healing bitters, calming Thai basil, chilled by coconut-water ice cubes. (Coconut water adds a whack of potassium and hydrates the body as well.) A gin and coconut elixir should always be served as a long drink: That is, in a tall glass, and it should run heavy on the gin and light on the seltzer and ice for maximum health benefits.

Coconut-water ice cubes (simply freeze unsweetened coconut water in an ice-cube tray overnight)

2 ounces (60 ml) botanical gin

1 ounce (30 ml) simple syrup (see page 155)

2 drops aromatic bitters (such as Bitter End Thai bitters or Angostura bitters)

1½ ounces (45 ml) seltzer water

Sprig of Thai basil (or regular basil)

Fill a tall glass with the coconut-water ice cubes. Pour the gin over them, followed by the simple syrup. Shake a couple drops of bitters into the glass and top with seltzer water (open a fresh bottle for maximum fizz!). Garnish with a single sprig of Thai basil, gently crushed to release its fragrant natural oils. This drink is especially soothing for a hot-weather hangover. ♋

Underberg Settler

Underberg is a powerfully healing herbal tonic that hails from Germany. Buy a bottle and you'll see that the slogan on the label reads, "After a good meal." True to its word, Underberg is a highly effective cure after overindulging in both food and drink. Serious imbibers keep a bottle or three handy for medicinal purposes—you never know when you might need it. Underberg can be enjoyed neat or mixed with tomato juice for a German take on the Bloody Mary. The Underberg Settler, created by world-famous Seattle mixologist Rocky Yeh, also features aromatic bitters, which were as commonplace on the shelves of early apothecaries as aspirin is today. Like Underberg itself, aromatic bitters add a punch to the dark rum that helps settle the belly and perk up the brain.

¾ ounces (22 ml) aromatic bitters

1 ounce (30 ml) dark rum

3 ounces (90 ml) sarsaparilla (or organic root beer)

Ice cubes (optional)

Combine all liquid ingredients in a mixing glass and stir. Add ice if desired, and strain into highball glasses. Rinse and repeat if necessary until that hangover disappears. ⌁

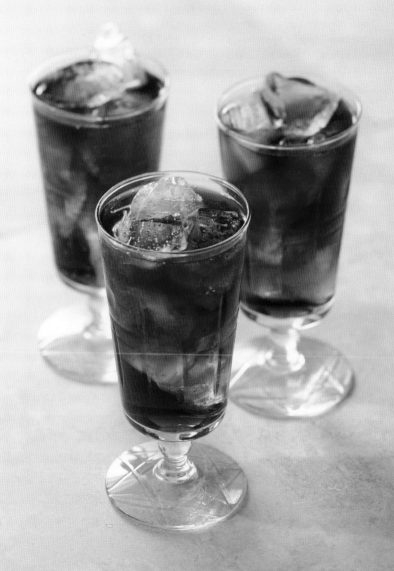

Aperol Fizz

There's nothing better than sitting down to a leisurely meal with all the trimmings: Lots of courses, wine pairings, and luscious desserts. Italian gourmands would agree: Historically, the citrusy Italian aperitif Aperol has been enjoyed before, during, and after lengthy meals to perk up appetites and ease digestion. Aperol gently raises the spirits as well as the appetite, especially when combined with aromatic bitters and fizzy water. It's just the thing if your spirits need a lift the day after a marathon meal with good friends. This historic cocktail was created to get tired bellies back on track, and it's so easy to make. Plus, since it's relatively low in alcohol, the Aperol Fizz is a sensible drink, so you'll be less likely to overindulge. It's the quick fix your digestive system needs!

---

2 ounces (60 ml) Aperol

Ice cubes

6 ounces (175 ml) sparkling natural mineral water (preferably one with a strong mineral flavor)

2 shakes Angostura bitters

Lemon zest twist

Add the Aperol to a Boston shaker and fill the shaker three-quarters full with ice cubes. Shake vigorously for twenty seconds. Add a few cubes of ice to a Collins glass; then strain the mixture slowly over the ice. Top the chilled Aperol with the sparkling mineral water; add bitters; garnish with the lemon zest twist; and prepare to be transported to an outdoor café in Italy. The Aperol Fizz is so light and refreshing, you have permission to go ahead and have another! ⤳

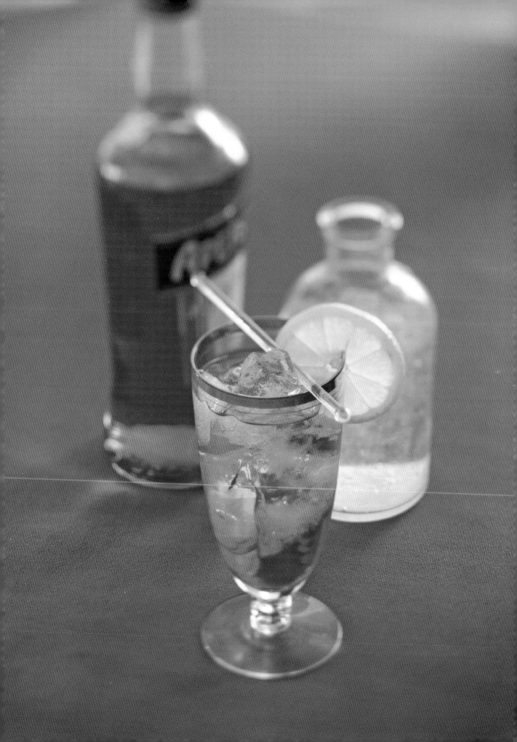

The Painkiller Prescriptive

The Painkiller Prescriptive has its origins at a beach bar known as the Soggy Dollar on the island of Jost Van Dyke in the British Virgin Islands. Medicinal preparations were available at this apothecary-cum-bar nearly every day during the winter and spring sailing seasons. If a sailor had spent the night in the grip of that demon, the "old black rum," a dose of this fruity prescriptive would be sure to cure him of the affliction—and fast. A distant cousin of the piña colada, the Painkiller both refreshes and heals: The citrus juices offer a wallop of immunity-boosting vitamin C, while the coconut provides potassium and adds creaminess and heft. Nutmeg, which has long been used to rouse the appetite, tops off the Painkiller—and, of course, the rum warms and soothes the sufferer's mind and body.

---

3 ounces (90 ml) navy-strength (over 90-proof) rum

1 ounce (30 ml) pineapple juice

1 ounce (30 ml) orange juice

1 ounce (30 ml) cream of coconut

Freshly grated nutmeg

Ice

Combine the rum, fruit juices, and cream of coconut in a Boston shaker. Then fill the shaker three-quarters full with ice and shake for thirty seconds or until the outside of the shaker becomes frosty. Resist the urge to slurp down immediately. Strain into a parfait glass filled with crushed ice, and top with freshly grated nutmeg. (Freshly grated nutmeg really is immeasurably better than pre-ground.) Serve with a straw, if desired. Anchors aweigh! ⌁

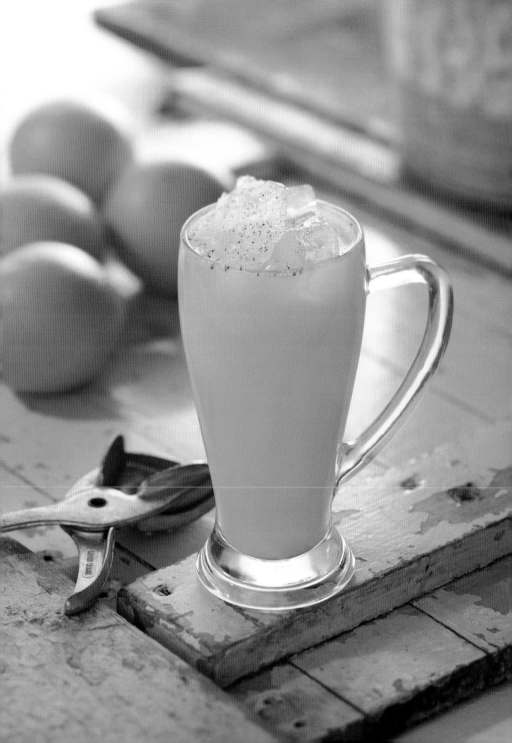

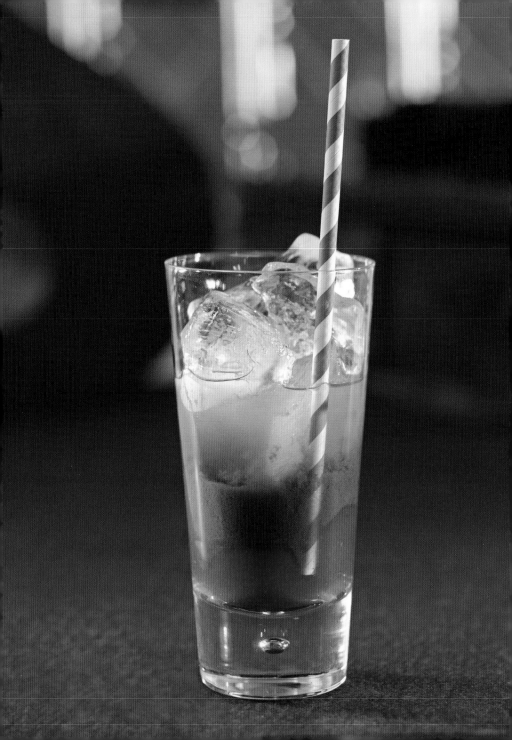

The Deep Healer

Chiles may set your heart racing and make you break out in a sweat with their fiery heat, but after eating them, you feel cleansed and purified, in both body and soul. Historically, pharmacies may have concocted products combining chile peppers with magnesium. When these ingredients were combined with grain alcohol and used either as an external salve or an internal elixir, they offered sufferers relief from painful ailments, such as lower back pain, muscle cramps, and fibromyalgia. Today, a chili-laden cocktail, such as The Deep Healer, is a great way to relieve headaches caused by overindulgence. Like the classic Bloody Mary, its tomato base is jam-packed with the antioxidant lycopene, and vodka gives it a heady kick, but the addition of onions, chiles, and leafy magnesium-rich green vegetables make it super-healthy, closer to a salad in a glass. A Deep Healer or two with a protein-packed brunch, such as a veggie omelette, will fix that pesky hangover in no time.

1 cup (250 g) tomato purée

½ cup (125 g) onion purée

¼ cup (65 g) hot chile paste

1 ounce (28 g) spinach, kale, or other dark leafy green

5 ounces (150 ml) vodka

Add all ingredients to a blender, and blend on regular speed until thoroughly combined. Serve over ice cubes in two tall glasses, and wait for the pain to evaporate. Serves two aching heads. ⟿

5 Relaxants and Toddies ⟩⟩
Drinks to Ease the Mind and Spirit

t was a wise man who first remarked, "You don't know what you've got 'til it's gone." And you can bet he was thinking about a good night's sleep when he said it. Most days, we take our shuteye for granted; we go to bed at night and get up in the morning with hardly a second thought. But anyone who's stayed up all night studying for exams in a coffee-fueled frenzy or sat up until dawn soothing a sick, feverish child knows that a full night of restful sleep is worth its proverbial weight in gold.

Restlessness and insomnia are nothing new, of course, so sleep preparations would have claimed an entire shelf of their own in historical apothecaries. The pharmacist was responsible for prescribing sedatives that could hasten sleep (and, ideally, still permit the patient to get out of bed the next morning). Sleep prescriptives in days of yore may have contained large quantities of opium or morphine, in addition to herbs suspended in alcohol, as well as other herbal ingredients. Obviously, it's best to skip the opiates and morphine these days, unless you're a celebrity with a bad track record—but there's still a range of natural sedatives that can safely be used to help you snooze.

Sedatives aren't just supposed to knock you out. They're meant to do several things that promote a "culture" of sleep, so to speak: They should relax the tense body, calm the distressed mind, alleviate stubborn pain, and generally inject a sense of serenity to the internal environment. Hot toddies, which combine spirits and herbs or other botanicals with boiling water, are easy-to-make cocktails that were traditionally used to warm the body thoroughly. Simply adding bitters and rum to a cup of hot tea has brought relief to the sleepless for hundreds of years—sailors of yore were especially fond of it. Today, it's hard to beat a hot toddy as a curative when sleep is the most important thing on your mind.

Other sedatives include the well-known cup of warm milk before bed—with the medicinal addition of a portion of Scotch whisky, for optimal results. Apothecaries from Germany's Black Forest region would prescribe a heady combination of blackberry brandy, tinctures made from indigenous herbs, and strong hot tea to help their patients get some shut-eye. In Mediterranean regions, a number of liquors are used as effective sedatives, such as the Italian digestif Amaro, cognac, and Calvados (or apple brandy). Post-prandial port or Madeira wine, consumed either neat or diluted with hot water, also facilitates healthy digestion, preventing belly-based sleep disturbances.

Plus, sedatives don't have to be sugary-sweet. Try adding a dash of liquor to steaming, savory soups or rich bouillons. Their strong flavors and stick-to-the-ribs consistency can nourish and relax. The same holds true for what's known as "pot likker," the vitamin-packed, green-tinged liquid that remains after cooking antioxidant-rich bitter greens, like collards, kale, turnip greens, or mustard greens. (According to legend, it's best when administered first thing in the morning along with a shot of rum—but it's certainly not a cure for the faint of heart.)

"The Scotsman's Slumber delivers a dose of Scotch whisky combined with piping-hot, wholesome beef bouillon—a surefire way to summon the sandman."

As you probably already know, synthetic sleeping pills can cause harmful side effects. Why not try herbs with natural sedative properties to help you get some rest? In the past, pharmacists might have prepared relaxing tinctures of herbs, preserved in a suspension of different liquors. Whether they're taken in combination with alcohol or not, chamomile, valerian root, and lavender can induce relaxation without resorting to chemicals, while peppermint and fennel can relieve ailments that keep you awake at night, like congested sinuses and indigestion. In this chapter, you'll find cocktails that use scores of tried-and-true herbal remedies for restlessness. The spicy-and-sweet *Mexican Sleep Cure* calls for correcting delicious (and easy to make) Mexican hot chocolate with mezcal to relieve wakefulness. *The Scotsman's Slumber* delivers a dose of Scotch whisky combined with piping-hot, wholesome beef bouillon—a surefire way to summon the sandman. While *The Cocktail Whisperer's Cold Cure #1001* may not be able to slay that dragon of a cold, it can help you get the sleep you need to shake it. The *Cold Cure*'s hot peppermint tea with Benedictine and healing Jamaican bitters help relieve body aches as well as blocked noses. *Herbal Sleep Punch* is a cool, gin-based cocktail that includes an infusion of healing herbs to rock you gently to sleep, while the *Sake Racer* combines Japanese sake and plum wine with a bit of gin. Take one, and you'll zoom off to sleep before you can even begin to count sheep. Or, if you're more of a minimalist, try one of the classic toddies featured in this chapter. Then sink into bed with a smile—restful sleep is just around the corner.

Note for the Reader:
All recipes make a single serving, unless otherwise indicated.
All herbs are fresh, unless otherwise indicated.

Sailor's Friend

This toddy is built with simple, honest materials that haven't changed much over the years: hot water, a large dose of spiced rum, and lemon—a trinity that can't help but hasten the old closed-eye relaxation. And we have the seamen of yore to thank for its popularity: Sailors whose watch was scheduled for the middle of the night would have to force themselves to sleep during the day, whether they liked it or not. This historically accurate toddy would have been a sailor's best friend when cold, misty nights made it difficult to get some shut-eye. Plus, honey has been used as an expectorant since Roman times. Today, it's still a powerful ally against scratchy sore throats and those pesky, chesty coughs that can keep you tossing and turning at night. Enjoy one an hour before bedtime.

Boiling water

3 ounces (90 ml) dark spiced rum

Honey, to taste

Lemon wheel

Preheat a mug by filling it with boiling water; discard the water after a few seconds. Add the rum to the mug and top with boiling water. Stir in honey to taste, and sip until sleep approaches off the ship's starboard side. Oh, and don't forget to float the lemon wheel on top of the toddy to stave off your chances of contracting scurvy. 〜

Mexican Sleep Cure

Pharmacologically speaking, alcohol-driven sedatives were originally created to treat individuals who were overwrought with stress. These sedatives relaxed the bodies and calmed the minds of the tense and jittery through the combination of hot, strong liquids and even stronger liquors. Common prescriptions from the pre-cocktail era included herbal or medicinal teas laced with fruit syrups and topped up with distilled alcohol for easier ingestion. Hot, bittersweet, chile-laden concoctions hailing from Mexico are also said to enhance repose and restfulness. Here, mezcal—a smoky, agave-based Mexican spirit—is added to a cup of spicy Mexican hot chocolate, and it's very effective when it comes to chasing the sandman. Skip the sleeping pills, and indulge in a cupful this evening.

3 ounces (90 ml) mezcal

1 cup (235 ml) Mexican "spicy" hot chocolate (combine ¾ cup [175 ml] of whole milk with a ¼ cup [60 ml] of heavy cream. Add ¼ pound [115 g] grated bittersweet chocolate. Heat slowly, do not boil, and whisk constantly until smooth. Add ½ teaspoon of cayenne pepper, and sugar to taste.)

½ teaspoon vanilla extract

Dark brown sugar, to taste

Prepare the hot chocolate. Preheat a mug by pouring boiling water into it; discard the water after a few seconds. Add the mezcal to the mug, followed by the hot chocolate, and then doctor it with the vanilla extract and sugar. Sip, and sleep is sure to follow. ⟿

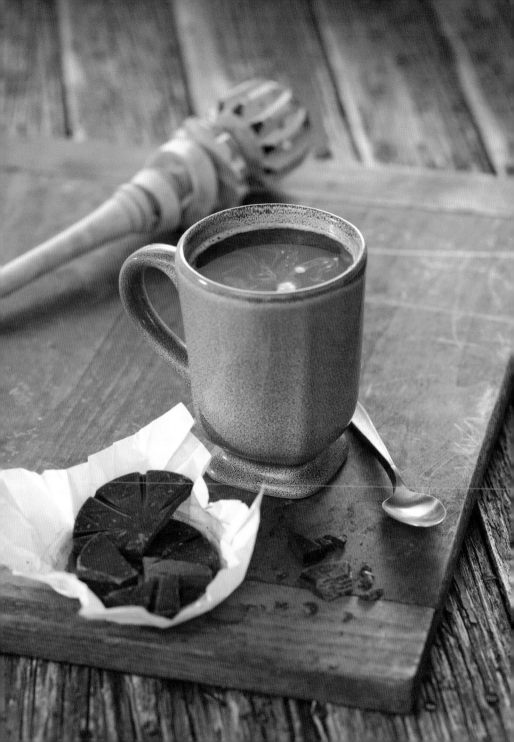

German Relaxation

We all know that restful sleep doesn't come easy, especially when you really need it. So it's no surprise that nearly every country in the world has developed its own remedies for wakefulness. In Germany, a teaspoon of distilled Alpine herbs suspended in a tonic made with wildflower honey and then added to a cup of hot water or tea is known to ease stress and to set tired eyelids fluttering. Made with dozens of herbs and spices—don't ask which ones, since the recipes for these tonics are usually guarded like state secrets. Today, many of these liqueurs are widely available outside of Deutschland, so they should be relatively easy to find. This simple recipe is just the ticket when it comes to combating restlessness and inducing relaxation.

3 ounces (90 ml) Alpine herbal elixir (such as Jägermeister)

6 ounces (175 ml) boiling water

1 ounce (30 ml) honey simple syrup (see page 157)

Preheat a mug by filling it with boiling water; discard the water after a few seconds. Add the Alpine herbal elixir to the mug, and top with more boiling water. Sweeten with the honey simple syrup, and you'll drift off to sleep dreaming of little goats frolicking on Alpine mountaintops. ☙

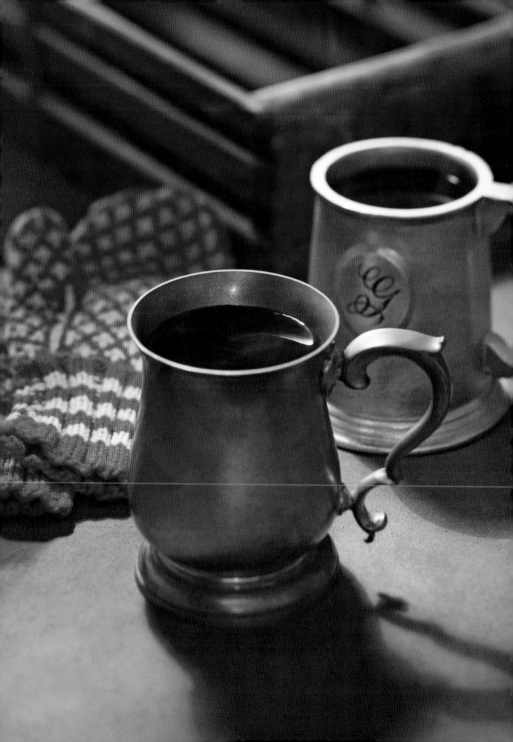

Rum Toddy for Restless Nights

Hot rum cocktails aren't just cold-weather cures. Sure, they're warming
and restorative, but they're also well-known curatives for sleeplessness.
Rum toddies like this one are simple to make and deliver powerful
healing to body and mind alike. This version calls for liberal dashes of
highly alcoholic, aromatic bitters, which are said to relieve anxiety and
insomnia by themselves. Here, they're added to a base of tannic black
tea that's been topped up with a hearty dose of rum and lemon—a marriage made in heaven—and then sweetened with honey. (If the caffeine
in tea keeps you up at night, just substitute with the decaf variety.)
Like a warm blanket, the gentle heat and fragrance from this toddy will
envelope you slowly, and sleep is sure to catch up with you fast.

---

3 ounces (90 ml) dark rum

6 ounces (175 ml) hot black
tea

Juice of one lemon

Several dashes of healing
bitters

One tablespoon (20 g) of
honey (or more to taste)

Prepare a pot of hot tea. Preheat a mug by filling
it with boiling water; discard the water after a few
seconds. Add the rum to the mug; then top it with
the tea. Mix in the lemon juice, add honey to taste,
as well as a dash or two (or three) of bitters. You
won't need to count sheep tonight! ➹

Scotsman's Slumber

Warm drinks made with Scotch whisky are tried-and-true ways for courting that elusive gnome named Sleep. That's because Scotch is a versatile healer: It's said to be effective against tension, restlessness, and even sleepwalking. In the heyday of apothecaries, high levels of stress probably contributed to insomnia. If the pharmacist could treat the stress, his patient would be more likely to get some shut-eye. And some things never change: Unfortunately, anxiety can still make bedtime an ordeal, but it'll ebb away after a few sips of this robust curative. Of course, Scotch is delicious—and remedial—when taken neat or on the rocks, but its unique, smoky flavor is also a great complement to savory beef broth. And this toddy is naturally caffeine-free, making it especially good at dimming the internal lights.

---

3 ounces (90 ml) Scotch whisky

6 ounces (175 ml) strong beef bouillon

Juice of ½ a lemon

Preheat a mug by filling it with boiling water; discard the water after a few seconds. Add the Scotch whisky to the mug and top it with the beef bouillon. Add a squeeze of lemon to the mixture, stir gently, and raise your mug to good health. As the Irish say, a good laugh and a long sleep are truly the best cures. ⟳

Cold Cure #1001

Colds can strike year-round, and when they do, they can keep you up at night—all night. It'd take magical powers beyond even the Cocktail Whisperer's understanding to actually cure a cold—but it's certainly possible to relieve its symptoms. Peppermint has analgesic qualities, which means it's known to ease cold-related pain like headaches. Peppermint infusions can also relieve ailments of the stomach, such as nausea, indigestion, and seasickness. It's also used in Bénédictine, one of the main ingredients in this insomnia-banishing drink. Be sure to crown your Cold Cure #1001 with Jamaican bitters, which are said to contain ingredients widely used in folk healing, such as allspice, ginger, and black pepper. Breathe deeply before taking a sip of this curative: If that pesky cold makes breathing feel like snorkeling with a drinking straw, a few whiffs of these aromas will alleviate congestion and speed snoozing.

12-ounce (355 ml) pot of hot peppermint tea

5 to 6 ounces (150 to 175 ml) Bénédictine

3 to 4 ounces (90 to 120 ml) sweet vermouth

10 drops Jamaican bitters

Prepare the pot of peppermint tea; then remove the teabags. Preheat two large mugs by filling them with boiling water; discard the water after a few seconds. Add the Bénédictine, followed by the vermouth, to the pot. Mix gently, and let the mixture sit for a few minutes. Add the bitters, pour into the mugs, and serve immediately. Inhale, soothing those grumpy sinuses. Serves two sniffling sufferers. ➷

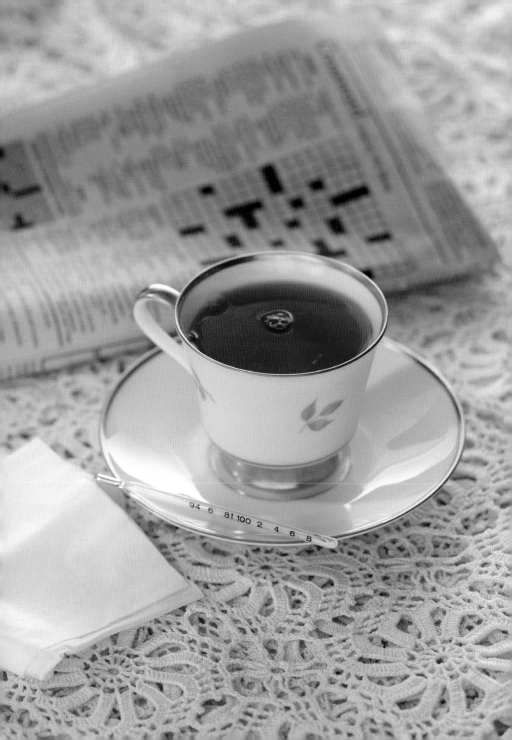

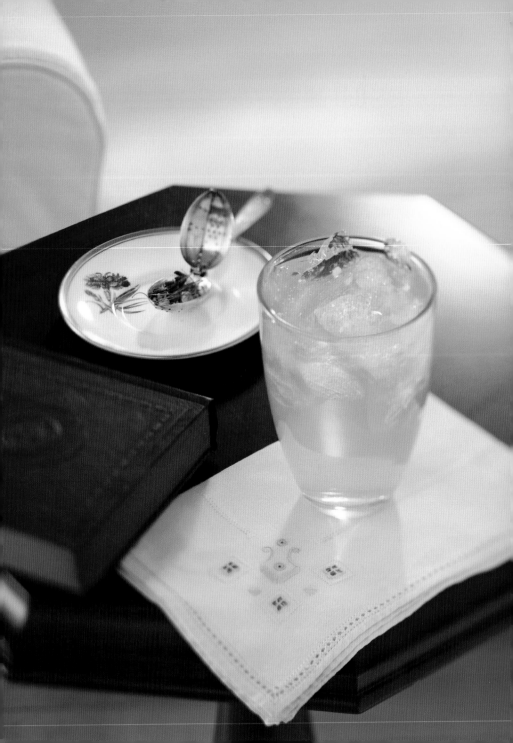

Herbal Sleep Punch

When it comes to curatives that enhance restful sleep, hot drinks aren't the only answer. In fact, I'm especially fond of cool liquids when sleep seems miles away. Toss out the sleeping pills: A punch made from herbal teas and botanical gin can relieve sleeplessness, even when it feels as if nothing could bring you a single step closer to the land of Nod. This cocktail combines infusions of herbs known to relax the sleep-deprived, and traditional apothecaries would have been well versed in their benefits. Chamomile, an anti-inflammatory, has been used as an antidote to anxiety for centuries, while lavender is said to gently ease irritating sleep disturbances. Fennel helps to keep digestion on track. A dose of botanical gin and lime juice bind the infusions together into a gentle tipple that will help turn off the lights for even the most dedicated insomniac.

---

1 teabag each chamomile tea, lavender tea, and fennel tea

Juice of 1 lime

Honey simple syrup (see page 157), to taste

3 ounces (90 ml) botanical gin

Ice

Infuse the teabags in 5 oz. (150 ml) hot water for at least an hour. When cool, pack a tall glass with ice. Pour the tea over the ice; add the lime juice, and sweeten to taste with the honey simple syrup. Finally, add the gin, and mix gently. G'night! ⌁

Sake Racer

If you're suffering from wakeful nights, enjoying sake—that is, Japanese rice wine—may encourage sleep to come knocking. Sake has a higher alcohol content than table wine, typically around 18 to 20 percent, but it's said to be gentler on the stomach than other forms of alcohol. Since it's packed with amino acids, it's even said to promote healthy skin when applied topically. (In creams and cosmetics, that is. Don't wash your face with it.) In addition to the warm sake—which shouldn't be heated over 140°F (60°C), by the way—the apothecary may suggest an infusion of healing, soothing herbs, along with a bit of botanical gin and a final touch of rich plum wine for sweetness. Combined, these ingredients can offer asylum from stubborn insomnia. Sayonara, sleeplessness!

6 ounces (175 ml) warm sake

3 ounces (90 ml) warm plum wine

2 ounces (60 ml) botanical gin

2 teaspoons healing herbs, such as ginseng, hops, caffeine-free green tea, or passion flower (add about ½ teaspoon of each to a mesh tea ball)

Preheat a mug by filling it with boiling water; discard the water after a few seconds. Pour the sake, plum wine, and gin in a large mug and stir gently; then let the tea ball steep in the mixture for at least five minutes. Remove the tea bag, and sip until sleep arrives like the moon over Mount Fuji. ⚘

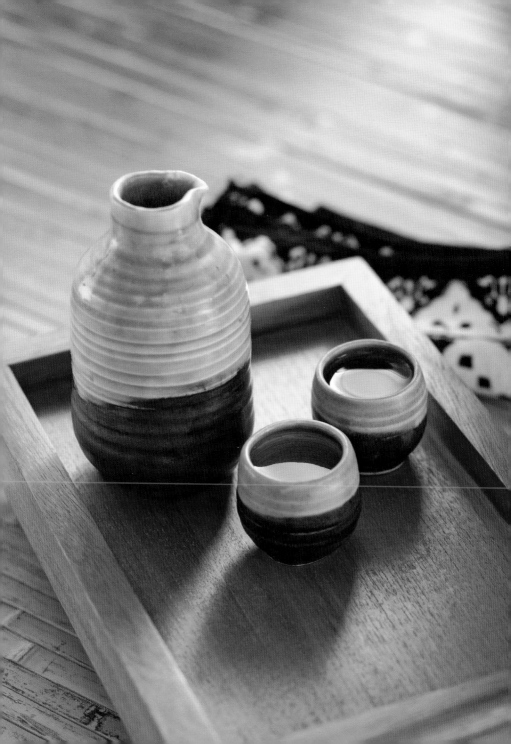

Nieuwpoort Elixir

Migraines, colds, and flus can chase sleep away fast, but rosemary may be able to help. This fragrant herb has been cultivated since ancient times, and for centuries it's been renowned for its potent antibacterial properties. (In fact, French hospitals used to burn it, along with juniper berries, to purify the air.) And humble rosemary offers many other health benefits that can speed snoozing: like chamomile, it contains anti-inflammatory properties; and peppermint is said to be good for pain relief. This Mediterranean herb is even more beguiling when combined with lime juice and genever, a juniper-flavored, herb- and spice-laden medicinal curative with roots in the Netherlands. This cocktail calls for fresh rosemary—whatever you do, don't substitute the dried version— suspended in ice cubes. As the cubes melt, the rosemary-infused water seeps into the drink, clearing pain-fogged heads before bedtime.

Rosemary water ice cubes (Place crushed rosemary leaves in an ice-cube tray and fill with filtered water and a few drops of simple syrup [see page 155]. Freeze overnight.)

3 ounces (90 ml) genever

4 ounces (120 ml) club soda

Lemon and orange twists

Several drops of Angostura bitters

Add several rosemary ice cubes to a Collins glass; then pour the genever and club soda over them. Mix gently, and finish with several drops of Angostura bitters. Garnish with the lemon and orange twists—then take three doses immediately. It's sure to relieve symptoms of malaise, letting you get the forty winks you long for. ↘

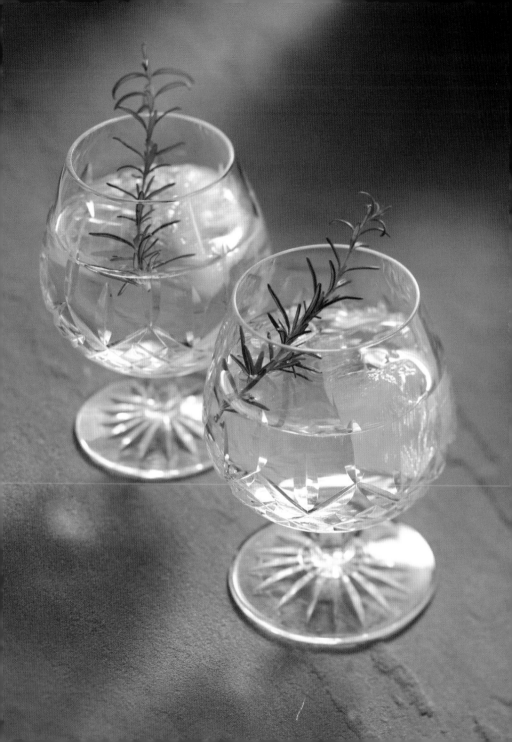

6 Painkilling Libations ❧
Ache-Soothing Analgesics

 e've all been there. You're just going about your day, and so far, everything's fine. Then, suddenly it hits: The headache from hell; a backache that makes you want to go straight back to bed; joint pain that just won't quit; or stomach cramps that leave you doubled over in agony. Now, you're not sure how you're going to get through the day in one piece. Aches and pains like these distract from daily life, and they can be frustrating, and even debilitating. Some people say that pain is just weakness leaving the body, and that may be true—but let's face it: It still hurts, darn it!

If you haven't got time for the pain, you're not alone. Your ancestors didn't have time for it, either. For hundreds of years, sufferers have been visiting apothecaries seeking solutions for pain of all sorts. Pharmacists prescribed different types of analgesics, in liquid, pill, or powdered form, as cures for body aches, headaches, toothaches, and even stomachaches. Early analgesics such as these often contained powerful concentrations of highly addictive, narcotic drugs, including heroin, morphine, and cocaine. When these narcotics were dissolved in alcohol and colored with vibrant dyes, the promise of a quick cure may have been too much for the pain-ridden to resist—but cures of this sort were far closer to quackery than they were to actual healing. Sometimes the cure truly was worse than the disease: Users of drugs like these ran a significant risk of becoming addicted to them, replacing illness with dependence. Fortunately, there were far less risky—and, arguably, more effective—curatives at the apothecary's disposal, ones that could offer competent relief from pain without causing addiction.

In theory, analgesics were created as a way to ease bodily pain during times of stress caused by injury or weakness—and it didn't hurt if they were able to calm the mind of the afflicted person as well. And, as any apothecary of days gone by would agree, many herbs, spices, fruits, and vegetables contain natural properties that can do both. But these delicate botanicals had to be preserved: Without refrigeration, many of them would have rotted, ruining their restorative properties—especially in warmer climates. That's where alcohol comes in. Suspending fragile botanicals in alcohol prevents rotting and can release their potential healing benefits. Blackberries, for example, have been used as analgesics for centuries—but how to preserve their painkilling power for months at a time? Combine them with high-proof spirits like vodka and brandy into a delicious infusion that'll last well into winter.

Of course, there are hundreds of natural remedies for easing pain. Celery juice has been used as an analgesic since Roman times, and today, it may be effective in relieving arthritis-related joint pain. Lavender and peppermint have offered relief from stress-induced headaches for centuries, while chamomile calms the entire body and, some say, quickly relieves menstrual pain. The herb lemon balm, a relative of peppermint, is also said to relieve tenacious body aches. Nutmeg is said to restore a wilting appetite, which can help ease the headaches and fatigue brought on by lack of food. Turmeric, garlic, ginger, chiles, poppy seeds, and anise also have longstanding reputations as painkillers.

"Sometimes simply drinking a fizzy glass of seltzer water can be a quick way to say 'no way' to pain."

When it comes to cocktails, though, easy-to-make tipples are surprisingly effective at chasing pain away. The combination of rum and cola—well known by sailors and other tipplers the world over—has been known to put a stop to headaches quickly. Rum relaxes the body, while cola provides an energizing (if less-than-healthy) sugar hit—as well as a dose of caffeine, just in case that headache is the result of coffee withdrawal. Cool liquids never do any harm when it comes to easing pain. Staying hydrated is a good way to prevent tiredness, headaches, and general sluggishness. Sometimes simply drinking a fizzy glass of seltzer water can be a quick way to say "no way" to pain.

These are just a few methods for easing pain that would have been at an apothecary's fingertips. This chapter includes plenty more delicious libations inspired by pharmacists of the past, such as a refreshing *Lemon Balm Gin and Tonic*: Using botanical gin and lemon balm-infused simple syrup, it's certain to whisk that headache away. Or, whip up an *Absinthe Frappé*, which combines powerfully soothing absinthe, fragrant mint, and plenty of crushed ice into a cooling concoction you can slurp up with a spoon. Craving something tropical? Reach for the *Cocktail Whisperer's Painkilling System #200*, which does what it says on the can: It knocks pain into oblivion through the judicious use of rum, citrus juices, coconut milk, and a dash of nutmeg. If you need something a bit warmer, try a *Green Tea Tonic*: It mixes gin with antioxidant-packed citrus, green tea, and Brazil nuts (yes, Brazil nuts) for a soothing analgesic that you can sip happily on a chilly evening. No time for pain? No problem.

Note for the Reader:
All recipes make a single serving, unless otherwise indicated.
All herbs are fresh, unless otherwise indicated.

Lemon Balm Gin and Tonic

When headaches strike, they can be frustrating, distracting, and even debilitating. Instead of reaching for synthetic painkillers, try a popular herbal cure that old-time pharmacists would've sworn by. Lemon balm, an herb related to mint, may be effective against a multitude of head-related maladies. Its lemon-scented leaves are used in the production of digestive liqueurs, such as amaro, Bénédictine, and chartreuse, and it boasts a long history of treating tension and stress, promoting refreshing sleep, and easing nervous conditions that may lead to headaches and even migraines. (Oddly, it can also act an effective mosquito repellent.) Lemon balm is often used in herbal teas, but here, it's infused in simple syrup and served up on ice with a generous dose of gin for a prescriptive take on the classic gin and tonic.

Ice

3 ounces (90 ml) botanical gin

2 tablespoons (30 ml) lemon balm simple syrup (see page 156)

¼ fresh lime, cut into chunks

Pack a tall glass with ice; then slowly pour the gin over the ice so it's well chilled. Add the lemon balm simple syrup and mix well. Top it with the tonic water and garnish with a lime chunk or two for an extra spritz of citrus. It's sure to clear the head and chase pesky headaches away. ➷

The Hartley Dodge Cocktail

*Bourbon or rye whiskey combined with sweet vermouth laced with
healing bitters can act as a powerful painkiller. Although this prescriptive resembles the classic Manhattan, adding muddled peach slices
to the mix adds a sweet, fresh, seasonal flavor thanks to the summery
stone fruit. And it's a fine balance: The key to this healing cocktail lies
in the right proportions of sweet, savory, and blatantly powerful. When
combined with the bottled-in-bond bourbon whiskey, the flavor of the
peaches becomes even more intense. "Bottled in bond," means the bourbon has been produced according to strict regulations, and it makes for
a tastier—and more effective—cocktail. Give it a try: The Hartley Dodge
has been known to conquer even the most tenacious aches and pains.*

---

3 slices fresh peach, plus
extra slices for garnish

3 ounces (90 ml) bonded
100-proof bourbon whiskey

1 ounce (30 ml) sweet
vermouth

4 dashes Fee Brothers
Whiskey Bitters

Ice cubes

Place the peach slices in a Boston shaker, and
muddle them. Add the bourbon and vermouth, and
continue to muddle so that the flavors are well
combined. Add the bitters and a handful of ice
cubes, and stir well. Strain into a Collins glass over
a large chunk of ice (larger pieces of ice are less
likely to dilute the drink). Garnish with an extra
slice or two of fresh peach. It's an analgesic that
can't help but take the edge off what ails you.

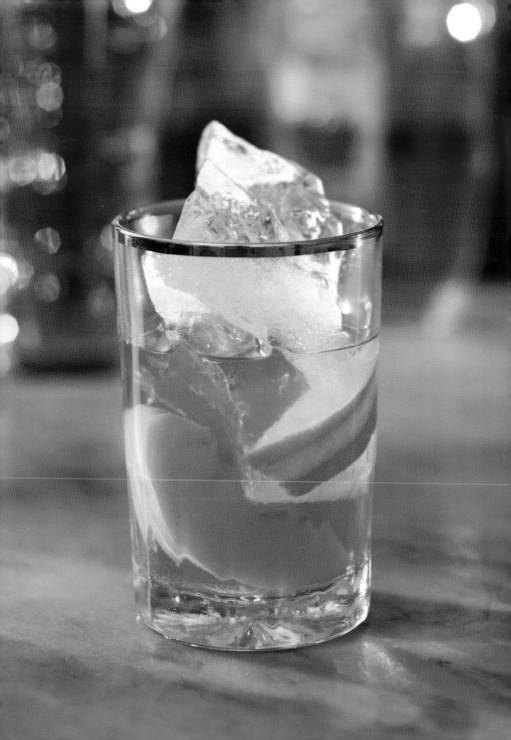

Blackberry Elixir

Berries are truly one of nature's super foods. Today, we know that they're high in antioxidants, jam-packed (no pun intended) with vitamin C, folic acid, and potassium, and may play a role in cancer prevention. But that wouldn't have surprised German apothecaries of days gone by. In Germany, blackberries and elderberries have been prized for their painkilling properties for hundreds of years. Blackberries contain salicylic acid, which has been known to act as an anodyne and may even protect against heart disease, while elderberries are said to combat pain resulting from rheumatism or traumatic injuries. Blackberry brandy, which apothecaries once prescribed as an able painkiller, is at the heart of this luscious elixir.

1 egg white

1 ounce (30 ml) lime juice

3 tablespoons (45 ml) berry vodka infusion (see page 157)

3 ounces (90 ml) botanical gin

Ice

Combine the egg white and lime juice in a Boston shaker, and shake without ice—a technique known as dry shaking—for one minute until the egg white stands up in fluffy peaks. Add 2 tablespoons (30 ml) of the berry infusion and the gin; then fill the shaker three-quarters full with ice, and shake for twenty seconds until well-combined. Place the remaining tablespoon of the berry infusion into a coupé glass, and pour the mixture over it. ⟲

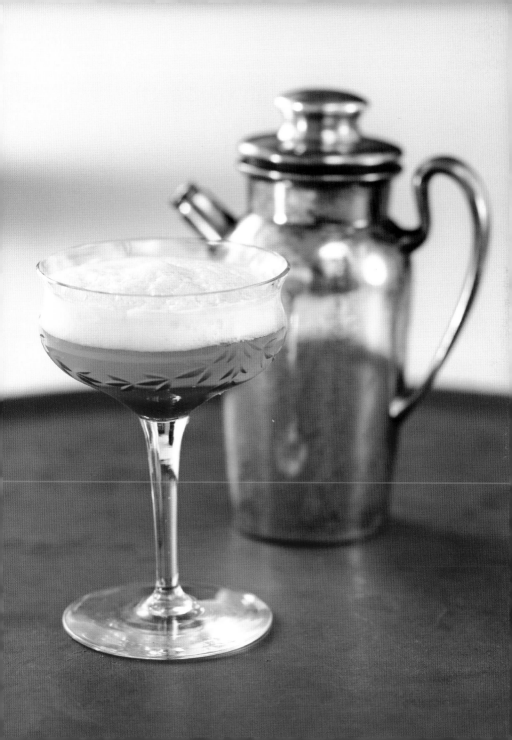

Cocktail Whisperer's Painkilling System #200

Sailors of the eighteenth and nineteenth centuries were well aware of rum's power as a painkiller. Here, fresh citrus juices balance out two types of rum, while orgeat syrup and a dash of coconut milk add sweetness and richness. Apothecaries would have known that a dash of nutmeg could act as an appetite stimulant. Here, a dash of the freshly grated spice reinvigorates tired taste buds with a flourish. My Painkilling System #200 is pretty powerful, though. In the wrong hands, the cure may be worse than the affliction. Stick to a single dose—or two, at most.

3 ounces (90 ml) dark rum

1 ounce (30 ml) 140-proof rum

1 tablespoon (15 ml) orgeat syrup

½ ounce (15 ml) sweetened coconut milk

2 ounces (60 ml) fresh pineapple juice

2 ounces (60 ml) freshly squeezed orange juice

2 ounces (60 ml) freshly squeezed grapefruit juice

Coconut ice cubes (see page 51)

4 dashes orange bitters

Freshly grated nutmeg

Fill a Boston shaker three-quarters full with plain ice. Combine all the liquid ingredients over the ice, and shake vigorously for twenty seconds. Fill a tall glass half full with crushed ice made from the coconut ice cubes, and strain the mixture into the glass. Garnish with a pineapple spear and a dusting of fresh nutmeg. Sip until pain free. ❧

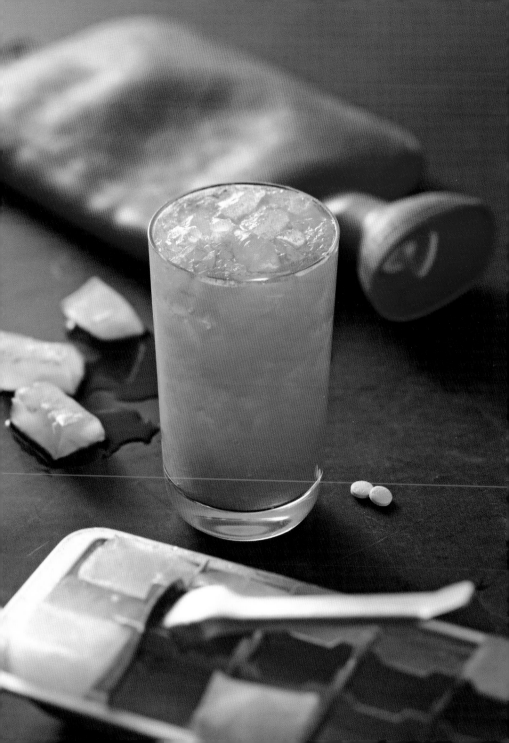

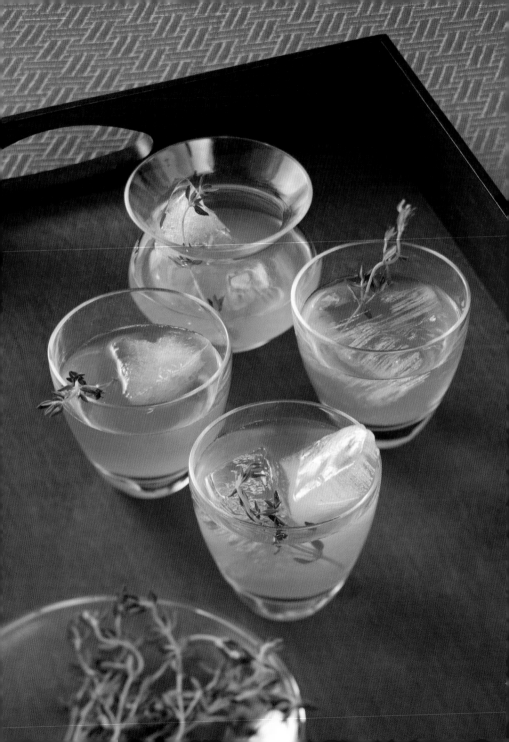

The Old Oak Tree Cocktail

Since time immemorial, the herb thyme has been prized for its stimulating, balancing properties. In healing preparations of old, pharmacists may have used it in a number of ways: as an antispasmodic, a digestive aid, a remedy for respiratory infections, and to promote healthy circulation and overall good health. Because it's highly antiseptic, early pharmacists would also have used thyme in a number of topical preparations, including salves and liniments. Like the Manhattan, The Old Oak Tree Cocktail combines vermouth with spirits and bitters, but this curative libation is rum-based, and it calls for a hit of fresh lime juice, which is a great complement to the rum. If you ask me, this restorative, analgesic cocktail can relieve the pain of just about any minor injury—from the inside out.

---

3 ounces (90ml) Rhum Vieux Agricole

1 ½ ounces (45 ml) cane sugar syrup

½ ounce (15 ml) sweet vermouth

3 to 4 dashes Angostura bitters

1 ½ ounces (45 ml) fresh lime juice

Sprig of fresh thyme

Ice

Combine the liquid ingredients in a Boston shaker. Fill the shaker three-quarters full with ice; then shake for twenty seconds. Strain the mixture into a rocks glass with one ice cube, and garnish with a sprig of thyme. Relax, sip, repeat, and let tension and body aches melt away. ᕯ

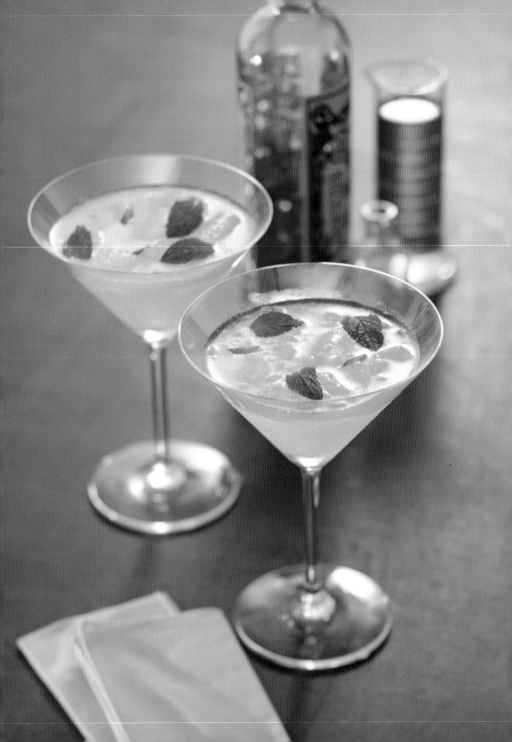

Absinthe Frappé

These days, when we think of frappés, we usually imagine high-octane, sugar-laden, iced-coffee drinks. Traditionally, though, a frappé is simply a liqueur poured over shaved ice—and it can be a delicious, refreshing treat. This take on the frappé privileges absinthe, which has a reputation for alleviating aches of all sorts due to its high alcohol level. Known as the Green Fairy because of the high chlorophyll levels of the botanicals originally used in its production—and because the psychoactive substances that were also present in them could make heavy drinkers hallucinate—absinthe is said to ease headaches and general malaise, and to soothe stomachs made ornery from exposure to spoiled food. Absinthe frappés have their roots in hot, humid New Orleans, where they were considered to be elegant, cooling potions that could be enjoyed all year.

---

2 ounces (60 ml) absinthe

½ ounce (15 ml) simple syrup (see page 155)

10 fresh mint leaves (plus extra for garnish)

3 ounces (90 ml) seltzer water

Crushed, pebble-sized ice

Combine the absinthe, simple syrup, and mint leaves in a large martini glass. Add the ice a spoonful at a time as you stir the absinthe mixture gently with a bar spoon, so that the glass becomes frosty. When the glass is nearly full, top with the seltzer water and stir gently. Tear a few mint leaves and strew them over the top of the drink. When nothing else will shift that truly dogged headache, this icy concoction can help. ↷

Green Tea Tonic

Genever, the botanical gin that hails from Holland and Belgium, has been used as a curative for over 500 years, and it's packed with healing ingredients, such as nutmeg, cinnamon, coriander, angelica, thistle, sweet orange peel, and grains of paradise. It's a natural match for citrus juices, like oranges and lemon—although in the early days of the apothecaries, citrus fruits were so exotic that you'd rarely catch a glimpse of them outside of the tropics. Nonetheless, pharmacists of yore may have prescribed a combination of fruits, spices, and grain-based spirits as a speedy antidote to pain. This warm tonic unites citrus, fresh ginger, green tea, and mineral-rich Brazil nuts, which are meant to reduce inflammation and relieve pain, into a gently warming prescription that eases all sorts of aches.

3 ounces (90 ml) genever

1 ounce (30 ml) freshly squeezed lemon juice

1 ounce (30 ml) freshly squeezed orange juice

1 tablespoon grated fresh ginger

1 tablespoon (15 g) powdered Brazil nuts

Warm green tea

Combine all ingredients in a small saucepan and warm over low heat until the ginger releases its perfume (about 10 minutes). Pour into teacups and serve. Relief is just a few minutes away. ✒

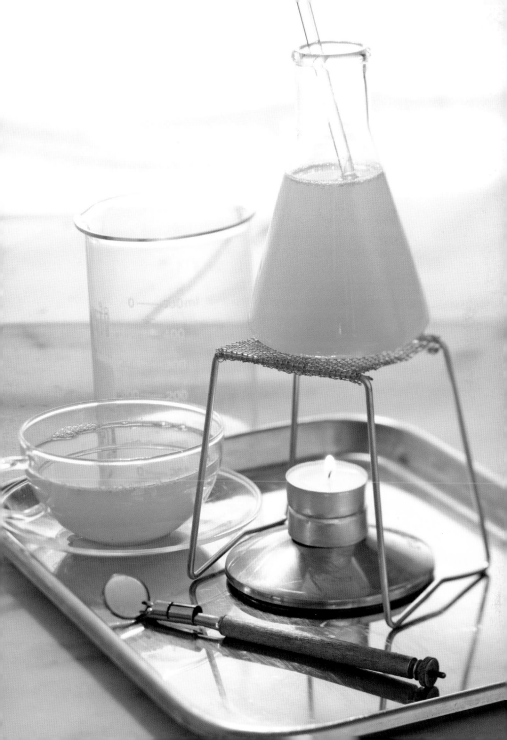

Coffee Soymilk Shake

Vegans, rejoice! Although there have been a lot of mixed messages about the health benefits of soy, it's safe to say that soy products can be consumed regularly as part of a balanced diet. It's been a staple of Asian diets for thousands of years, and today, soy milk is still a great source of protein. It may help restore and repair damaged muscle tissue, and soy milk might be able to soothe pain that stems from other sources, such as premenstrual tension. So there's no reason why you shouldn't enjoy a soymilk shake after a long workout, or if you're simply feeling achy. A soymilk shake like this one, made with coffee liqueur and overproof rum, can help fight pain, especially pain in the extremities, such as fingers and toes. (Is that due to the healing powers of soy, or the rum? Try one and find out.)

---

6 ounces (175 ml) soy milk

1 ounce (30 ml) coffee liqueur

2 ounces (60 ml) overproof rum

Ice

Combine the soy milk, coffee liqueur, rum, and ice in a blender. Process until smooth; pour into a tall glass, and serve with a straw or two. Remember to sip slowly, or you'll bring on another kind of pain: the dreaded ice cream headache. ➤

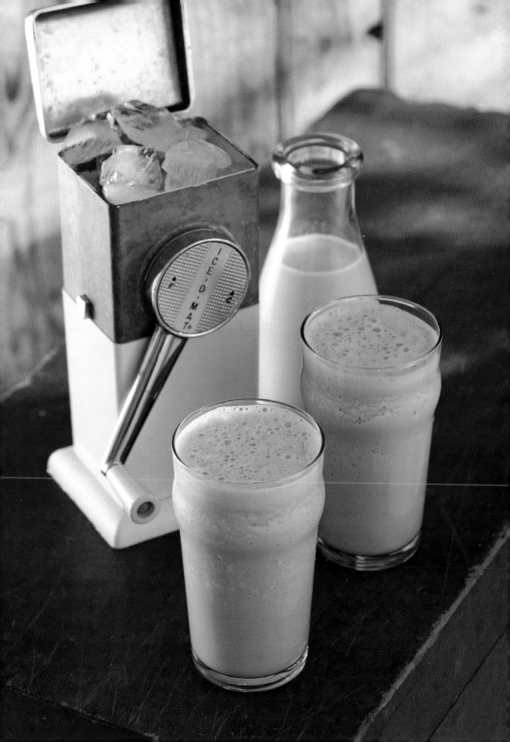

Watermelon Martini

We all know that a balanced diet is a huge part of good health, and
that it's important to get our five daily servings of fruits and vegetables.
But it's also possible that some fruits, such as oranges, peaches, cherries,
grapefruit, and watermelon may actually be able to alleviate pain in
addition to being, well, simply good for you. Aim to eat fruits of many
different colors; those with deep, vibrant hues, like watermelon, tend to
pack an especially substantial wallop of antioxidants. Cocktails that
include watermelon, like this refreshing Watermelon Martini, can help to
relieve headaches and back pain. Inspired by apothecaries of yesteryear,
who would have preserved concoctions of fruits and spices in preservative spirits, it combines freshly crushed watermelon with aromatic,
curative vermouth and citrus-tinged botanical gin. It's a deeply delicious
curative that may assuage aches gently and quickly.

½ ounce (15 ml) dry
vermouth

3 ounces (90 ml) botanical
gin

2 ounces (60 ml) puréed
watermelon

Lemon zest twist

Ice

Wash a cocktail shaker with the vermouth; then
pour it out (into your mouth, if you like!). Fill
the shaker one-quarter full with ice; then add
the gin and puréed watermelon. Stir, strain into
a coupé glass, and garnish with a lemon zest
twist. Prost!

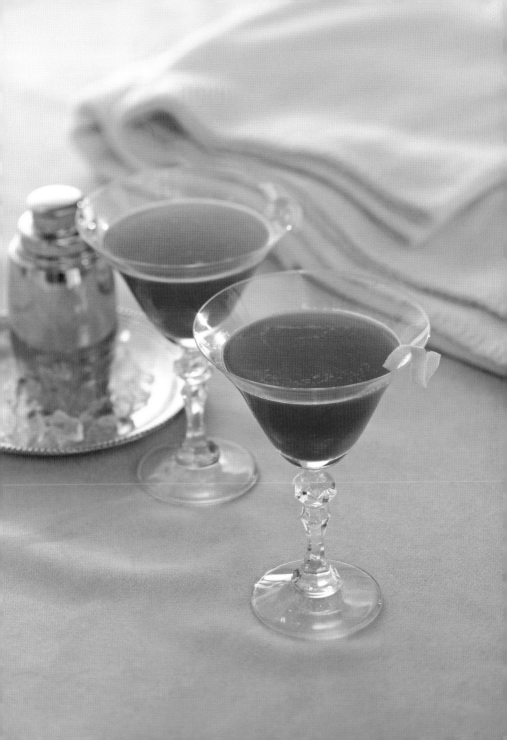

Pain-Proof Garden Elixir

If you're suffering from joint pain due to arthritis, natural remedies may help—and one particularly powerful remedy comes straight from the garden. Fresh vegetables can assist in the treatment of arthritis, especially those with vibrant colors: think spinach, broccoli, tomatoes, and carrots. The antioxidants in these vegetables help reduce joint swelling and inflammation, and the more you eat of them, the better. Here, a variety of veggies are lightly steamed, then puréed into a concentrated "soup" that's packed with pain-fighting nutrients. Adding vodka turns the healthy mixture into a miniature cocktail that can be served Russian-style: that is, well chilled, and doled out in shot glasses. (Talk about literally drinking to your health.) If you enjoy a classic Bloody Mary, you'll love this savory, nutritious libation.

---

10 cups (710 to 900 g) fresh vegetables, such as lightly-steamed broccoli, asparagus, tomatoes, cabbage, and cauliflower, lightly steamed and puréed in a blender

2 cups (475 ml) vodka

Combine the puréed vegetables and the vodka in the blender, and continue to purée until the mixture is smooth. Chill in the fridge; then administer in shot glasses (or other small glasses). Raise your glass high and drink to pain-free joints. 🗲

Sweet Sherry Elixir

The essential oil of the herb oregano is another powerful ally when it comes to fighting pain. It's said to alleviate arthritis pain as well as headaches of all sorts and descriptions, and in some cultures, is even used to relieve sore throats. But you don't need to use very much of this intensely flavored herb to heal deeply: Just a drop or two will do the trick. And, curiously, oregano's flavor is a good complement to sweet sherry. Happily, sherry isn't just for medicinal purposes: It's an important ingredient in cocktails, and, of course, it's delicious on its own. When the two are combined, the result is a sweet earthiness that's intensely relaxing. (In the past, the pharmacist might even have prepared a batch of oregano-based bitters especially for this curative tipple.) Today, this simple cocktail is still a winner.

---

3 ounces (90 ml) sweet Sherry

1 drop (and no more than 1 drop!) oil of oregano

Pour the sherry into a brandy snifter (or small juice glass). Then, using a medicine dropper (or just extreme care), add a single drop of oil of oregano to the sherry. Sniff deeply, inhaling the potent, earthy aroma. Then pick up your glass and put the aspirin away! ➥

Twisted Mint Julep (Cocktail Whisperer Style)

It's difficult to sing the praises of mint too loudly. In addition to perking up congested sinuses and calming sour stomachs, mint is also said to be effective against throbbing headaches. So there's no reason to confine mint juleps to the Kentucky Derby. In this healing cocktail, a twist on the original mint julep, mint's essential oils act as a foil to strong liquor: Mint cools the body while the liquor warms it. Speaking of liquor, I'm a big fan of using rye whiskey in my mint juleps. If you ask me, bourbon is just too sweet! Plus, the rye from which rye whiskey is made may possess more healing qualities: It's said, surprisingly, to contain a whole host of antioxidants, and is even reputed to prevent gallstones. That's good enough for me.

½ ounce (15 ml) absinthe

10 fresh mint leaves, plus
  1 sprig for garnish

3 ounces (90 ml) rye whiskey

Dark muscovado sugar

Crushed ice

Chill a Collins glass by filling it with ice water; then pour it out after a few seconds. Pour the absinthe into the glass, swirl it around, and pour it out (or simply drink it, if you like). Put half of the mint leaves in the bottom of the glass with a very small amount of ice, and add about ¼ teaspoon of sugar. Muddle the mint until it begins to release its essential oil. Add one ounce (30 ml) of whiskey, another ¼ teaspoon of sugar, more ice, and a couple more mint leaves, and continue to muddle. The glass should become frosty as you work. Repeat until you've used all the whiskey and mint, and the glass is nearly full. Garnish with a sprig of mint. Pain doesn't stand a chance against this cooling curative. ➤

7 Mood Enhancers

Good Cheer in a Glass

 bad night's sleep can bring it on. Stubbing your toe—yet again—can do it. Thinking about that visit to the dentist on Monday morning will definitely cause it to flare up, and missing your bus is a surefire way to provoke it.

We're talking about bad moods, and they can be triggered by just about anything—and nothing. Some days seem to set a series of unfortunate events into motion, ones that would try the patience of any Pollyanna. And before you know it, you find yourself snapping at co-workers and glaring at passersby. Other times, you simply wake up on the wrong side of the proverbial bed—several mornings in a row. The question is, how do you snap out of it?

Apothecaries would have been asked that very question. Before the advent of powerful, synthetic antidepressants in the mid-twentieth century, sufferers would have turned to herbal cures for relief from stormy moods. Pharmacists had a variety of remedies at their disposal. Teas made from valerian root or chamomile could relieve anxiety and irritation, and could help the patient fall into a restorative sleep that would ease peevishness. The natural oils in sage can promote a sense of calm and content, which could have taken the nervous edge off the stressed and the restless. St. John's wort is still used today in supplement form to balance negative moods. Spices like turmeric were thought to have anti-inflammatory properties, and may have been able to alleviate joint pain (and liven up the libido, too).

"Before the advent of powerful, synthetic antidepressants in the mid-twentieth century, sufferers would have turned to herbal cures for relief from stormy moods."

And of course, alcohol was recommended as an antidote to glum moods, and as a way to restore flagging energy. The authors of an 1826 pharmaceutical textbook published in London claim that "[a]rdent spirits … increase the general excitement, communicate additional energy to the muscular fibres, strengthen the stomach, and exhilarate the mind." Although the authors do insist that these spirits shouldn't be taken in "immoderate doses," you can be sure that very few of the apothecary's patients would've resisted a healing dose of sherry or brandy merely to "calm the nerves," that is. Using alcohol would've helped preserve the healing power of the pharmacist's botanicals, too. It truly was essential for medicinal purposes.

Healing potions require more than herbs and spirits, though. Many mood-enhancing apothecary concoctions might have included preparations that used sparkling water. After all, many apothecaries and pharmacies also featured built-in soda fountains, which attracted customers of all ages. Carbonated water was popular in medicinal preparations because of its lively, refreshing bubbles, which could help the patient believe that the ingredients were doing their healing work. Sparkling curatives were—and perhaps are—simply more convincing. And besides, a fizzy drink gives concentrated herbal flavors a lift, making them far more palatable (and decreasing the alcohol level of the prescriptive, too). Plus, even though adding sparkling water to alcoholic curatives dilutes them, its effervescence makes them seem extra potent, since the carbonation in it lets your bloodstream absorb the alcohol quickly. Simple cocktails of rum, juices, bitters, and fizzy water became an easy way for the pharmacist's patient to soothe upset stomachs, relax edgy nerves, and ingest a healthy dose of vitamin C—all at once.

That's why many of the cocktails in this chapter use cheap-and-cheerful soda water or seltzer water as a main ingredient, such as the *Milk Thistle Spritz*, which mixes the purifying herb with a dose of Italian aperol into a cocktail that's both detoxifying and delicious. The *Les Héretiers Curative* is a classic combination of cane-sugar rum with bitters, coconut water and—you guessed it—bitters: Inspired by all things tropical, it's a refreshing way to relax both body and mind after a long day. *The Bosphorus Cocktail* uses seltzer water to enliven a unique mixture of carrot juice, Turkish raki, and turmeric. Even its bright-orange color is cheerful, and since turmeric is reputed to be an effective aphrodisiac, it won't be long before you chuck that bad mood and replace it with thoughts of amore. But if fizzy drinks aren't your thing, try a *Flemington Cocktail*, which combines aromatic sage with Scotch whisky, sweet vermouth, and luscious stone fruits. Or, mix up a batch of *Sherry Cherry Cobblers*: In it, that traditional cure-all, sherry, is laced with rum-soaked cherries for a digestif that's certain to put a smile on your face.

Of course, good overall health is probably the best way to ensure stable moods and a positive attitude. The Cocktail Whisperer's mood-enhancing cocktails are best enjoyed in moderation, and in the company of good friends. Try to avoid overindulging, or you'll have to head back to the apothecary for a hangover cure. The moral of the story: As a wise man once said, "Eat your bread with gladness, and drink your wine with a merry heart."

Note for the Reader:

All recipes make a single serving, unless otherwise indicated.
All herbs are fresh, unless otherwise indicated.

Milk Thistle Spritz

Set firmly in the early ages of the apothecary, this healing spritz derives its benefits from the curative herb milk thistle, which has been renowned as a "liver tonic" for hundreds of years. Milk thistle promotes digestive health and helps the liver eliminate toxins. In fact, it may both prevent and repair liver damage. And when the liver is doing its job well, the entire body feels better. During the apothecary era, ingesting spoiled food often couldn't be helped, so pharmacists would be called upon to provide antidotes to such illnesses. That's where milk thistle comes in: By cleansing the body deeply, it lightens both the patient's body and mind. This cocktail also includes the Italian digestif aperol, which makes it a delicious way to finish a meal.

1 tablespoon (15 ml) milk thistle powder

2 ounces (60 ml) aperol or Campari

4 ounces (120 ml) white rum

2 ounces (60 ml) freshly squeezed lemon juice

2 ounces (60 ml) simple syrup (see page 155)

2 to 3 ounces (60 to 90 ml) seltzer water

4 drops Peychaud's bitters

Ice

Combine all the ingredients except the seltzer water and bitters over a few handfuls of ice in a Boston shaker. Shake for a few seconds until well combined.

Divide the mixture between two Collins glasses; then top each with the seltzer water, and add two dashes of bitters per glass. Serve, imbibe, and prepare to feel refreshed and renewed. Serves 2.

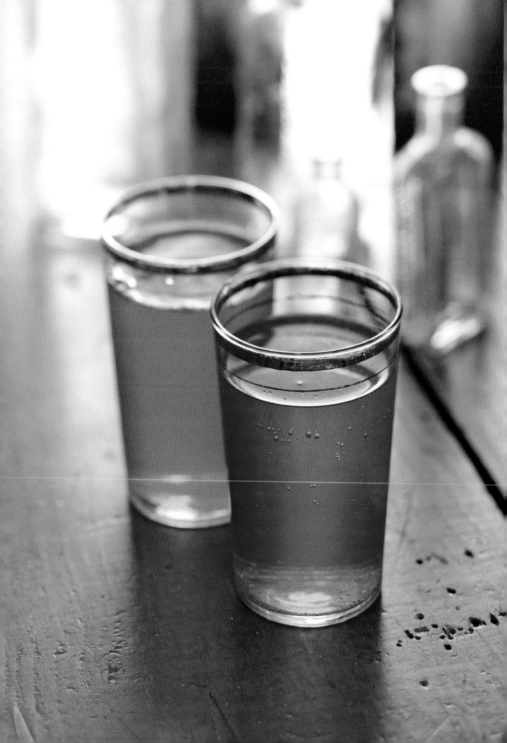

Flemington Cocktail

If you're in need of a pick-me-up, skip the caffeine-laden coffee and sugary snacks. Instead, get inspired by apothecaries of years past, who would have known that sage could help their patients feel calmer, more relaxed, and contented. Sage's Latin name, salvia officinalis, is derived from the verb salvere, meaning "to save" or "to heal," and pharmacists of old would have used it in liquid-driven tonics to help lift gloomy moods. Plus, it's reputed to have anti-inflammatory properties and to boost brain function and enhance memory. The scent of clary sage has often been recommended for relieving symptoms of stress and anxiety. When it comes to good cheer, it's just what the apothecary ordered.

---

3 tablespoons (60 g) muddled stone fruits (peaches, plums, or nectarines)

1 ounce (30 ml) honey simple syrup (see page 157)

3 ounces (90 ml) Scotch whisky

½ ounce (15 ml) sweet vermouth

Few dashes Angostura bitters

1 ounce (30 ml) freshly squeezed lemon juice

1 large fresh sage leaf, chiffonaded (that is, rolled up like a cigar and finely sliced across the grain)

Muddle the stone fruit in the bottom of a Boston shaker. Add the honey simple syrup, Scotch whisky, sweet vermouth, bitters, and lemon juice, and shake for twenty seconds until combined. Strain the mixture into a martini glass, and garnish with the chiffonaded sage leaf. Sip slowly until the dark clouds start to lift. ➤

Les Héritiers Curative

Back in the day, apothecaries in the Caribbean knew just what to do if a patient complained of feeling heavyhearted or glum. They'd prescribe a hearty dose of their favorite curative, Rhum Agricole. Made from cane sugar, this overproof rum would've acted as a preservative for delicate herbs and spices, and it might have given the patient a much-needed buzz at the end of an interminable—and possibly expensive—curative session. Rum takes pride of place in the Les Héritiers Cocktail, alongside healing bitters and fizzy water. The bubbles in effervescent water were thought to facilitate cures by quickly getting them into the bloodstream and promoting circulation. Today, drinks that feature sparkling water are still wonderfully refreshing. Les héritiers means "the princes" in French, and you're sure to feel like one after a dose of this delicious prescriptive.

3 ounces (90 ml) Rhum Agricole

1 ounce (30 ml) cane-sugar syrup

1 ounce (30 ml) coconut water

2 ounces (60 ml) seltzer water

2 dashes bitters

Ice

Combine all the liquid ingredients except the bitters in a cocktail shaker. Add a few handfuls of ice, then the bitters. Taste, and add another dash or two of bitters to taste, if you like. Strain the mixture into a coupé glass, and serve. Relax, sip, and repeat, and let that cranky mood drift away. ↷

Chartreuse Curative

Saffron has been used in Ayurvedic medicine and Asian and Med-iterranean cooking for thousands of years. Derived from the crocus flower, this precious spice has been praised for its healing qualities: It's reputed to be an antiseptic, antidepressant, antioxidant, digestive aid, and anti-convulsion restorative. And it's been used in the production of herbal liqueurs like Chartreuse, something French imbibers enjoy as an after-dinner drink. Of course, saffron is astronomically expensive, but never fear: As with most good things, a little goes a long way. This mood-lifting prescriptive combines top-quality chartreuse with vermouth and egg white for a colorful, frothy little cocktail that'll brighten up even the greyest day. Top it off with a thread or two of saffron as a nod to Chartreuse's luscious color.

---

3 ounces (90 ml) Chartreuse VEP

1 ounce (30 ml) dry vermouth

1 egg white

2 to 3 saffron threads

Ice

Add the chartreuse, vermouth, and egg white to a Boston Shaker; then fill the shaker three-quarters full with ice. Shake vigorously for twenty seconds until frothy. Strain the mixture into a coupé glass, and garnish with the saffron. Then sit back and watch sinking spirits rise. ➶

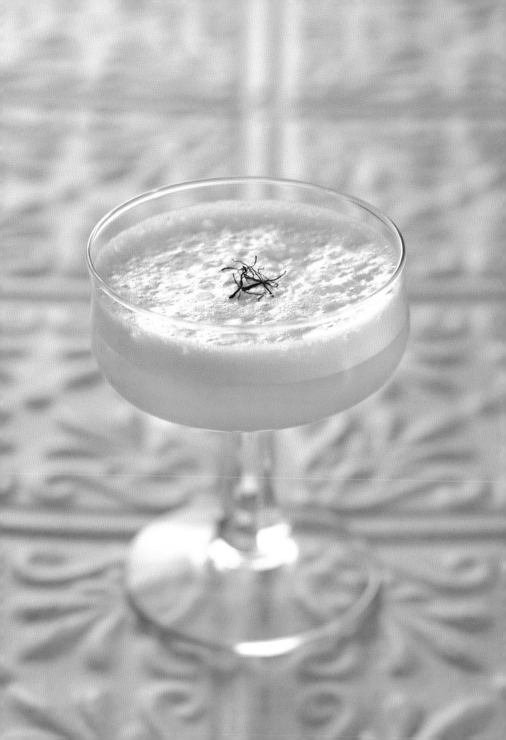

Campari and Soda Water Quick Fix

Campari, that ultra-powerful Italian digestive, has an incredible red hue due to its unique mixture of citrus, herbs, and spices. The medicinal tipple is often mixed with a dose of freshly squeezed lemon juice to ward off vitamin C deficiencies and other nutrition-related maladies. It's often taken neat, but with the addition of a few ounces of carbonated water, Campari becomes more than just an after-dinner treat: It's transformed into a prescriptive that can affect the spirit as well as the body. Sparkling water delivers the scent of the aromatic, therapeutic herbs straight into the patient's nose, relieving his stomachache, headache, and grumpy mood all at once. Aperol, another bright-red, Italian-made herbal liqueur, can be substituted for the Campari in this easy recipe: It's used to liven up diners' moods and whet their appetites before big meals.

---

4 ounces (120 ml) Campari

3 ounces (90 ml) club soda (with an added pinch of salt)

Orange zest twist

Ice

Add a handful of ice cubes to a Collins glass. Pour the bright-red Campari over the ice and top with the club soda. Garnish with a flamed orange zest twist (pinch the zest firmly and hold it behind a lit match to release the citrusy oils). Breathe deeply: The scent will perk you up before you've even taken a sip. ↷

Chinese Iced Tea with Star Anise

Strangely enough, star anise isn't related to aniseed—although the two herbs share a distinctive, licorice flavor, and both are used to alleviate upset stomachs and freshen breath. Star anise is frequently used in traditional Chinese medicine to warm the body and stimulate circulation. It's also said to possess antibacterial and antifungal qualities, and is often added to hot tea to relieve persistent colds, coughs, and other flu symptoms. This curative, an Asian-influenced take on the classic iced tea, is a great way to lift flagging spirits and refresh hot, tired bodies on a sultry summer day. Anise, ginger, and lemon are flavorful complements to one another, while antioxidant-rich Chinese black tea may be good for heart health. Top it off with botanical gin, and you've got a cocktail that's as tasty as it is healing.

1 small pot (about 2 cups [475 ml]) iced Chinese black tea

2 pods Chinese star anise

4 tablespoons (60 ml) ginger simple syrup (see page 156)

3 ounces (90 ml) freshly squeezed lemon juice

6 ounces (175 ml) botanical gin

Sprig of fresh mint for garnish

Ice

Brew the pot of Chinese black tea; then let it cool. Add the star anise, ginger simple syrup, lemon juice, and gin to the pot, and mix well. Pack two Collins glasses with ice; then fill them with the iced tea, and garnish each glass with fresh mint. Serves 2 tired tipplers. ⟋

The Bosphorus Cocktail

Turmeric is one of the many spices used in amari, which are bitter-tasting, digestive liqueurs popular in Italy. Turmeric is packed with healing properties. It's said to be an anti-inflammatory, an expectorant, and may alleviate a number of digestive disorders—and, according to traditional Chinese medicine, turmeric may be useful for easing depression. Surprisingly, it's also reputed to be a powerful aphrodisiac. This prescriptive delivers a healthy wallop of turmeric suspended in nutrient-rich carrot juice laced with the Turkish liqueur raki. Rose-infused simple syrup adds a hint of sweetness to take the bitter edge off the raki, and a splash of soda water makes the Bosphorus Cocktail remarkably refreshing and stimulating. Oh, and it might even offer a certain kind of lift to those who suffer from, ahem, certain deficiencies when it comes to matters of the boudoir.

---

2 ounces (60 ml) raki

4 ounces (120 ml) carrot juice

1 teaspoon turmeric

2 tablespoons (30 ml) rose-infused simple syrup (see page 157)

3 ounces (90 ml) soda water

Ice

Add the raki, carrot juice, turmeric, and rose-infused simple syrup to a Boston Shaker. Shake well until combined (about twenty seconds). Place one large ice cube in a rocks glass, and strain the mixture into the glass over the ice. Then top with soda water, and sip for a much-needed lift to both body and mind. ❧

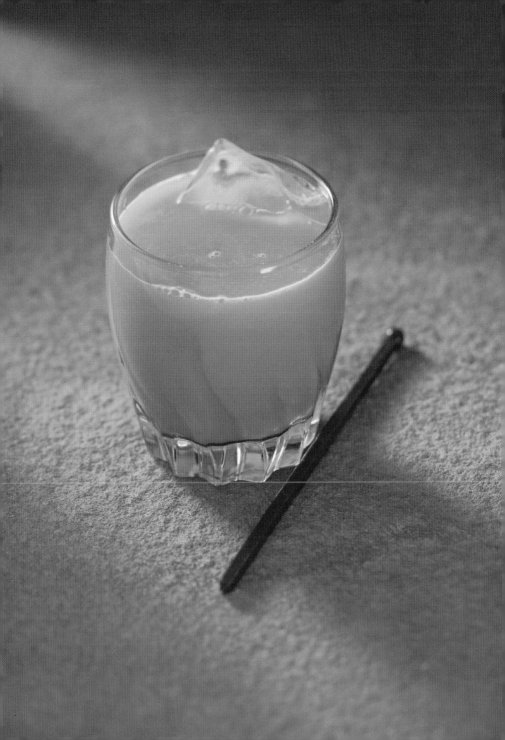

The Enlightener

The Mexican spirit mezcal is a potent beast. Made from the agave plant, which is said to be sacred in Mexican culture, it has a pale-yellow color, sports a distinctively smoky aroma, and is usually served neat. Apothecaries of old might have suggested a slug of this firewater to those whose love lives were drooping, since it's reputed to lift the libido. Although some say its smoky scent and flavor make it a less versatile spirit than, say, tequila, it's easy to use it to great effect in a cocktail that's a distant relative of the margarita. The Enlightener brightens up mezcal with sweet agave syrup, a trio of citrus juices, and a dash of fizzy water, creating a crisp, fragrant, vitamin C-laced tipple. Palate-stimulating Mexican bitters top off this memorable slurp. It's a refreshing route to good cheer, Cocktail Whisperer-style.

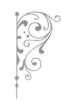

---

3 ounces (90 ml) mezcal

2 ounces (60 ml) agave syrup

1 ounce (30 ml) freshly squeezed orange juice

1 ounce (30 ml) freshly squeezed grapefruit juice

1 ounce (30 ml) freshly squeezed lime juice

2 ounces (60 ml) seltzer water

4 drops Mexican bitters

Lime wheel for garnish

Add the mezcal, agave syrup, and fruit juices to a Boston shaker filled three-quarters full with ice. Shake for about twenty seconds, until the vessel is frosty. Strain into a coupé glass, and top with the seltzer water and then the bitters. Pop the lime wheel over the edge of the glass for garnish. Lift your glass, and say goodbye to the blues. ➤

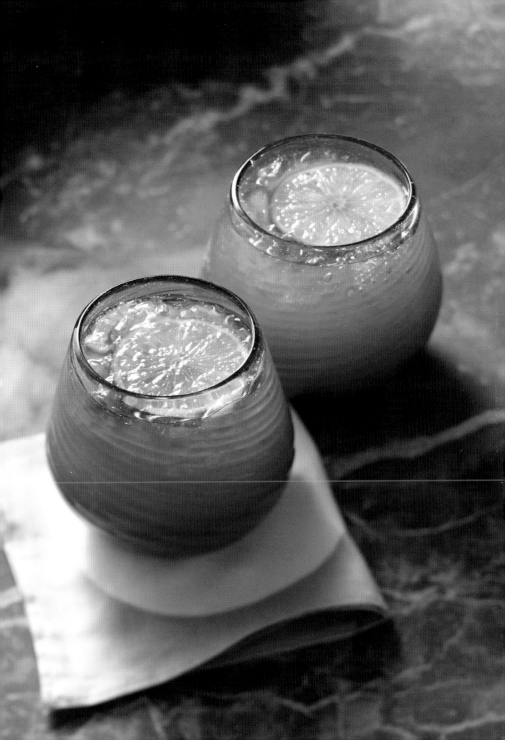

Cardamom and Rum Elixir

Cardamom is frequently used in Asian cuisine, and it also appears regularly in Ayurvedic preparations and traditional Chinese medicine. It promotes the flow of chi, or life-energy, which means it's warming and invigorating, and it's reputed to help rid the body of harmful impurities. Cardamom is also said to stimulate the nervous system, reduce inflammation, and act as an expectorant. Early pharmacists in America would have used cardamom and other exotic spices extensively—if they could get them—when treating patients with flu symptoms. In this invigorating cocktail, the purifying spice is steeped in simple syrup and combined with cane-sugar rum, then bathed in fizzy water. The result is a flavorful, powerful curative that's as tasty as it is healing. It's sure to boost the spirits and brush the cobwebs away.

2 ounces (60 ml) Rhum Agricole

½ ounce (15 ml) cardamom simple syrup (see page 156)

4 ounces (120 ml) seltzer water

2 dashes Angostura bitters

Ice

Combine the rum and cardamom simple syrup in a Boston shaker filled three-quarters full with ice. Shake until combined and chilled (about fifteen seconds). Place one ice cube in a short rocks glass; then strain the mixture over the ice. Top with the seltzer water and add the bitters. Sip slowly, and let the ice melt into the cocktail. By the time your glass is empty, that melancholy mood will be ancient history. ⟋⟍

Sherry Cherry Cobbler

In days of yore, pharmacists often prescribed sherry as a nerve tonic, or as an antidote to insomnia. (Because it was considered medicinal, even teetotalers would happily take a glass or two!) It's still a delicious way to finish a good meal, and adding a dash of seltzer to sherry makes it that much more uplifting. In eighteenth-century England, the fizzy mixture had a reputation for curing foul moods. Sherry "punches" made with stone fruits are a delicious way to nip that bad mood in the bud, especially if it was brought on by a touch of indigestion. Oh, and here's another reason to treat yourself to a Sherry Cherry Cobbler: Stone fruits like cherries are antioxidant-rich, while sherry may have some of the same heart-healthy properties that red wine does.

¼ cup (60 g) rum-cured cherries (store-bought, if you can find them: Alternatively, chop 1 cup [155 g] fresh, pitted cherries, and steep in 1 cup [235 ml] rum in a stainless steel bowl for one week before use. Store in the refrigerator.)

2 ounces (60 ml) fino (dry) sherry

2 ounces (60 ml) sweet sherry

1 teaspoon Peychaud's bitters

4 ounces (120 ml) seltzer water

Ice

Place the cherries in a Boston shaker, and add the sherries. Muddle the cherries, then add the bitters and fill the cocktail shaker three-quarters full with ice. Shake for twenty seconds; then strain the mixture into a coupé glass, and top with the seltzer water. (Grab a spoon and eat the muddled cherries that remain in the cocktail shaker, if you like!) Serve, sip, and float away on a cherry-flavored cloud. ↱

Doctor Livesey's Cocktail

In the heyday of apothecaries, medicines usually tasted terrible and weren't often prettied up through the addition of sweeteners or coloring as they are today. So, as the song goes, a spoonful of ginger could truly help the medicine go down. Alternatively, ginger itself could be used as medicine, since it's said to be an effective cure for a variety of ailments, including headaches, motion sickness, fatigue, and pregnancy-related nausea. Ginger, a close relative of turmeric and cardamom, appears in many forms, including powders, syrups, suspensions, tonics, salves, and infusions, and traditional Chinese medicine is rife with the healing root. Combining ginger with hot punches or beer is a classic way to use the root as a curative, as sailors of yesteryear would have known. Named after the honorable doctor in Robert Louis Stevenson's classic, Treasure Island, *this cocktail matches ginger beer with its natural partner, rum, into a tipple that rouses the mood and washes the doldrums away.*

3 ounces (90 ml) dark rum

4 ounces (120 ml) ginger beer (non-alcoholic)

Lime wedge for garnish

Ice

Fill a Collins glass with ice cubes. Pour the ginger beer over the ice; then float the dark rum on top. Garnish with a lime wedge to keep scurvy at bay. Drink slowly, and let good cheer fill your sails.

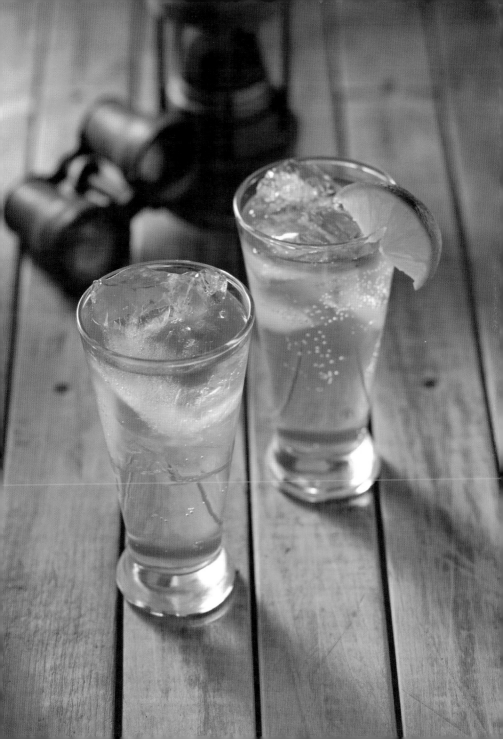

Mead Refresher

Everyone knows that royal jelly, which is produced by worker bees and fed to their hive-mates, is an important curative in health preparations. But raw—that is, unprocessed —honey is also deeply curative, and what's more, the distillation of spirits using raw honey is an ancient, well-regarded technique. Honey has been used medicinally at least since ancient Egyptian civilization, and beverages produced from honey, such as mead, have been enjoyed since time immemorial. "Mead is good," wrote the nineteenth-century German herbalist, Sebastian Kneipp, because it "increases the hunger, stimulates digestion, purifies and strengthens the stomach, and frees the body of bad substances." He wasn't wrong: Raw honey may possess antibacterial qualities and is said to promote weight loss, reduce cholesterol, and relieve symptoms of intestinal disorders. This bubbly cocktail combines sweet mead with tart, refreshing lemonade and a dash of fizzy water into a prescriptive that is sure to cheer and heal at the same time.

6 ounces (175 ml) mead

6 ounces (175 ml) fresh lemonade

4 dashes of aromatic bitters (any kind: it's up to you)

4 ounces (120 ml) seltzer water

Combine the mead, lemonade, and bitters in a mixing glass or pitcher. Stir to combine, and pour into four short glasses. Top each glass with about 1 ounce (30 ml) of seltzer water. Serves 4. So it won't be long before you and three friends feel like the proverbial bee's knees. ❧

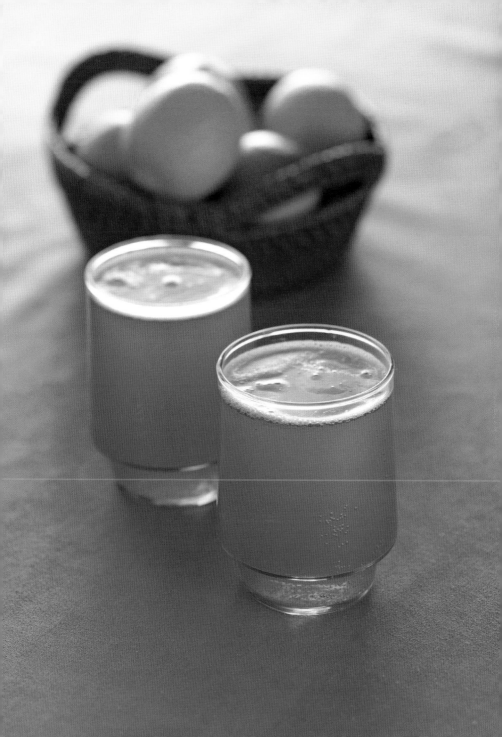

Honey Healer

In Germany, certain herb-based liqueurs are produced with enzyme-rich honey from the Yucatan Peninsula in Mexico to offset the liqueurs' acerbic bitters. This rich, darkly colored honey is a great healer. Raw honey has been said to alleviate the symptoms of seasonal allergies when consumed regularly, and may be good for digestive ailments like colitis. In Ayurvedic medicine, too, honey is highly valued—it's reputed to be one of the most powerful substances for promoting good health in general. And honey can sweeten the spirit as well as the body: Suspending it in alcohol and combining it with black or herbal tea and plenty of ice makes it a highly refreshing mood enhancer. The honey, rum, and German herbal spirits in this tall cocktail weave an enchanting spell— one that never fails to relax, re-animate, and restore.

---

12 ounces (355 ml) cool black tea

4 tablespoons (80 g) raw honey

6 ounces (175 ml) navy-strength (over 90-proof) rum

3 ounces (90 ml) German herbal liqueur

Ice

Prepare the tea; stir in the honey; and let the mixture cool. Pack two glasses with crushed ice, and divide the rum and the herbal liqueur between them. Top each glass with the honey-sweetened tea. Stir, taste, adjust the sweetness if necessary, and say guten Morgen to a great mood. ⟲

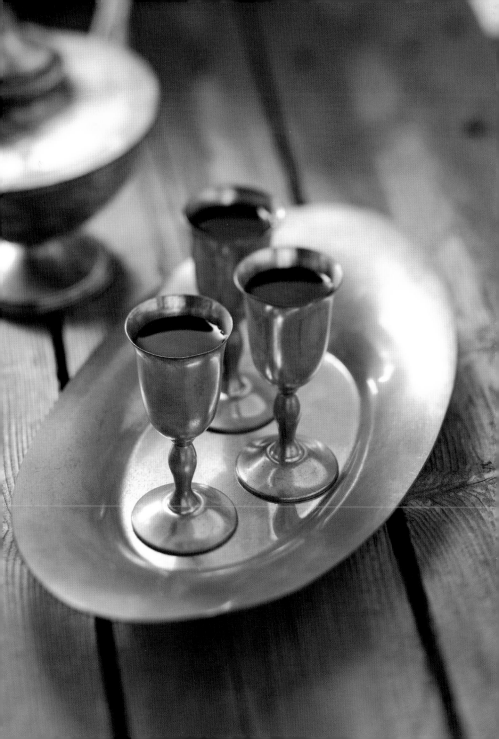

The Ail and Cure Swizzle

The Ail and Cure, a cousin of Doctor Livesey's Cocktail, was created by cocktail connoisseur Christopher James, head bartender at the four-star Ryland Inn in Whitehouse, New Jersey. Chris says, "I can envision this cocktail being sipped during a beautiful day, on an island, by someone who might have a bit of a bellyache. Ginger beer was used medicinally in the Caribbean in the eighteenth and nineteenth centuries, since ginger was especially good for relieving stomach pain. Angostura bitters were developed by a German army doctor, Dr. Ben Siegert, in Venezuela to aid his troops in the digestion of their food. And we all know Caribbean rum can very well cure all the imagined ills that ail you! With the first sip of this drink, as you inhale the soothing scent of the aromatic mint garnish, I'm sure you will be transported to this special place I've imagined—and I'm positive your bellyache or bad mood will subside."

2 ounces (60 ml) dark rum

¾ ounce (22 ml) orgeat

1 ounce (30 ml) fresh lime juice

2 healthy dashes of Angostura bitters

4 ounces (120 ml) ginger beer (non-alcoholic)

Rock candy swizzle stick

Sprig of fresh mint

Ice

Fill a tall pilsner glass three-quarters full with crushed ice. Pour the first four ingredients over the ice, and mix well with the rock candy swizzle stick. Top with the ginger beer, and gently swizzle again for a second or two to combine. Top with more crushed ice, and garnish with a sprig of mint. Grumpy moods will disappear over the horizon.

Syrups and Infusions ❧

An incomparable collection of syrups, purées, and infusions to add to your repertoire.

Simple Syrup

Add **1 cup (235 ml) of boiling water** to **1 cup (200 g) of bar sugar or caster sugar** and mix until sugar has dissolved. Let the mixture cool. Keep refrigerated in an airtight container for up to a month.

Cardamom Simple Syrup

Make a batch of simple syrup (above) and pour it into a medium-sized bowl. Add **2 to 3 crushed cardamom pods** to the mixture and let it cool. Cover the bowl with plastic wrap, place it in the refrigerator, and let the pods steep in the syrup for 1 to 2 days. Remove the cardamom pods, and keep refrigerated in an airtight container for up to a month.

Root Tea Simple Syrup

Combine **4 ounces (120 ml) of organic root tea liqueur** with **½ cup (100 g) bar sugar** and **1 cup (235 ml) boiling water**. When the sugar has dissolved, let the mixture cool, and keep refrigerated in an airtight container for up to a month.

Healing Herb Simple Syrup

Make a batch of simple syrup (above) and pour it into a medium-sized bowl. Place the **assorted herbs** into a cheesecloth bag and tie tightly with string. Submerge the cheesecloth bag in the simple syrup—let the string hang outside of the bowl, like a teabag, for easy removal. Cover the bowl with plastic wrap, place it in the refrigerator, and let the herbs steep in the syrup for 1 to 2 days. Remove the cheesecloth bag of herbs before using. Keep refrigerated in an airtight container for up to a month.

Fennel Simple Syrup

Make a batch of simple syrup (above) and pour it into a medium-sized bowl. Add **¼ cup (16 g) chopped fresh fennel** to the mixture and let it cool. Cover the bowl with plastic wrap, place it in the refrigerator, and let the fennel steep in the syrup for 1 to 2 days. Strain before using, and keep refrigerated in an airtight container for up to a month.

Shrubb Simple Syrup

First, juice **12 limes**, and grate **two 6-inch (15 cm) ginger roots**. Combine **2 cups (400 g) of bar sugar or caster sugar** with the lime juice in a small saucepan; then add the grated ginger and **½-cup (120 ml) apple cider vinegar**, and combine. Warm over a low heat until the sugar is completely dissolved. (This may take a while, so please be patient.) Let the mixture cool then cover, with plastic wrap and refrigerate for 1 day. Strain the ginger out of the mixture before using. Keep refrigerated in an airtight container for up to a month—or until the mixture feels fizzy on the tongue when tasted.

Lemon Balm Simple Syrup

Make a **batch of simple syrup** (page 155) and pour it into a medium-sized bowl. Add **10 to 12 torn lemon balm leaves** to the mixture and let it cool. Cover the bowl with plastic wrap, place it in the refrigerator, and let the lemon balm steep in the syrup for 1 to 2 days. Strain before using, and add up to 2 ounces (60 ml) of botanical gin as a preservative, if desired. Keep refrigerated in an airtight container for up to a month.

Cardamom, Clove, and Rose Simple Syrup

Make a **batch of simple syrup** (page 155) and pour it into a medium-sized bowl. Add **1 tablespoon (15 ml) of rosewater** to the syrup. Then place **1 teaspoon of whole cloves** and **2 to 3 crushed cardamom pods** into a cheesecloth bag and tie tightly with string. Submerge the cheesecloth bag in the simple syrup—let the string hang outside of the bowl, like a teabag, for easy removal. Cover the bowl with plastic wrap, place it in the refrigerator, and let the spices steep in the syrup for 1 to 2 days. Remove the cheesecloth bag before using. Keep refrigerated in an airtight container for up to a month.

Ginger Syrup

Add **1 cup (200 g) of sugar** to 1 cup (235 ml) of boiling water. Grate **8 oz. of ginger root** into the mixture, and then let it stand in the refrigerator for a couple of days. Strain, and now you have ginger syrup. Keep refrigerated in an airtight container for up to a month.

Roasted Tomato Puree

Preheat the oven to 400°F (200°C, or gas mark 6). Line a baking tray with parchment paper. Toss **1 pound (455 g) of grape tomatoes** with **2 tablespoons (30 ml) of olive oil** and a **dash of salt**. Arrange the tomatoes on the baking tray, and roast for half an hour. Then turn the heat down to 250°F (120°C, or gas mark ½) and slow-cook them until melted, about 3 hours. (Keep an eye on them. If they start to burn, turn the heat down, but be patient. You want the tomatoes to melt, not burn.) When the tomatoes are cool enough to handle, puree them either in a food processor or with a mortar and pestle to make a relatively smooth liquid. Add **2 to 4 tablespoons (30 to 60 g) of horseradish** (freshly-grated is best, if you can get it), **several squeezes of fresh lemon juice**, and a **dash of celery salt**. Store in the refrigerator for up to 3 days.

Honey Simple Syrup

Add **1 cup (235 ml) of boiling water** to **1 cup (340 g) of honey** and mix until honey has dissolved. Let the mixture cool. Keep refrigerated in an airtight container for up to a month.

Rose-Infused Simple Syrup

Place **2 to 3 organic red rose petals** into a cheesecloth bag and tie tightly with string **(use organic rose petals only)**. Pour **1 cup (235 ml) simple syrup** into a small bowl, then submerge the cheesecloth bag in bowl. Cover it with plastic wrap, and store in the refrigerator overnight. Remove the cheesecloth bag before using. Alternatively, combine **1 tablespoon (15 ml) of rosewater (be sure to use the edible kind!)** with **1 cup (235 ml) of simple syrup** in a small bowl, and store in the refrigerator overnight before using. Keep refrigerated in an airtight container for up to a month.

Berry Vodka Infusion

1 cup (145 g) of elderberries in **½ cup (120 ml) of blackberry brandy**. Add **6 ounces (175 ml) of vodka** and combine well. Cover with plastic wrap. Keep the mixture in the refrigerator for 2 days, then purée the mixture in a blender or food processor, and strain it through cheesecloth. Keep refrigerated in an airtight container: It'll last for months.

Acknowledgments

In keeping with the standard practices of saying thank you to those who have influenced me to become an author, I must give pause. There are so many to thank, but a few who really helped me keep the lights on at night. My wife, Julie, successfully encouraged me to do what I love, and find where my passion lay as so many had tried over the years, yet failed miserably.

There is the 501c3, Wild River Review and Joy Stocke who allowed me to establish the Wild Table blog when I was unpublished and unknown. She guides me to this day in my quest to become a better and more succinct writer.

My food writing teachers, Alan Richman and Andy Smith, could have just as easily said for me to stick to banking. (They didn't)

There are the people like Laura Baddish at the Baddish Group and the Steven Grasse at Quaker City Mercantile who saw my talent, as well as Foodista, DrinkUpNY, Beverage Media Group, and *Total Food Service* magazine.

There are the brands that I write for, who keep me in vast quantities of samples, which help me dream in new flavor combinations. My talent for mixology comes from being a former chef. The dreams of flavors through scratch cooking are firmly rooted in the kitchens that I spent much of my time working.

My fresh pasta business in Charleston, South Carolina, during the 1980s, although ultimately a financial failure, set me up for the emotional success of *Apothecary Cocktails*.

To Served Raw Magazine, which considered me the magazine's cocktail whisperer back in 2010, when no one had even heard of my name, I say thank you...

To all those who have taught me the value of listening and allowed me a seat at their table, I say thank you. People such as Chef Anthony Bucco and my bar mentor Christopher James; and the friendship of Gary Regan, who taught me the merits of a finger-stirred Negroni.

But none of this would have been possible without the email that I received out of the blue, from Jill Alexander asking me if I wanted to submit some writing samples for a potential book on apothecary cocktails. To this end, I say thank you.

About the Author

Warren Bobrow is the food and drink editor of the 501c3 nonprofit Wild River Review, in Princeton, New Jersey. He was one of twelve journalists worldwide, and the only one from the United States, to participate in the Fête de la Gastronomie, held September 2012, in the Burgundy region of France. Warren is the former owner and cofounder of Olde Charleston Pasta in Charleston, South Carolina, while cooking at the Primerose House and Tavern (also in Charleston). He has published over 300 articles on everything from cocktail mixology to restaurant reviews to travel articles. Warren was # 30 in *Saveur* magazine's 100 in 2010 for his writing about the humble tuna melt. He also writes for the "Fabulous Beekman 1802 Boys" as their cocktail writer (Klaus, the Soused Gnome). You may find Warren on the Web at www.cocktailwhisperer.com

Index